Sports Injuries in the Military

Editor

BRETT D. OWENS

CLINICS IN
SPORTS MEDICINE

www.sportsmed.theclinics.com

Consulting Editor
MARK D. MILLER

October 2014 • Volume 33 • Number 4

ELSEVIER

1600 John F. Kennedy Boulevard • Suite 1800 • Philadelphia, Pennsylvania, 19103-2899

http://www.theclinics.com

CLINICS IN SPORTS MEDICINE Volume 33, Number 4
October 2014 ISSN 0278-5919, ISBN-13: 978-0-323-31172-4

Editor: Jennifer Flynn-Briggs
Developmental Editor: Donald Mumford

Photocopying

Single photocopies of single articles may be made for personal use as allowed by national copyright laws. Permission of the Publisher and payment of a fee is required for all other photocopying, including multiple or systematic copying, copying for advertising or promotional purposes, resale, and all forms of document delivery. Special rates are available for educational institutions that wish to make photocopies for non-profit educational classroom use. For information on how to seek permission visit www.elsevier.com/permissions or call: (+44) 1865 843830 (UK)/(+1) 215 239 3804 (USA).

Derivative Works

Subscribers may reproduce tables of contents or prepare lists of articles including abstracts for internal circulation within their institutions. Permission of the Publisher is required for resale or distribution outside the institution. Permission of the Publisher is required for all other derivative works, including compilations and translations (please consult www.elsevier.com/permissions).

Electronic Storage or Usage

Permission of the Publisher is required to store or use electronically any material contained in this periodical, including any article or part of an article (please consult www.elsevier.com/permissions). Except as outlined above, no part of this publication may be reproduced, stored in a retrieval system or transmitted in any form or by any means, electronic, mechanical, photocopying, recording or otherwise, without prior written permission of the Publisher.

Notice

No responsibility is assumed by the Publisher for any injury and/or damage to persons or property as a matter of products liability, negligence or otherwise, or from any use or operation of any methods, products, instructions or ideas contained in the material herein. Because of rapid advances in the medical sciences, in particular, independent verification of diagnoses and drug dosages should be made.

Although all advertising material is expected to conform to ethical (medical) standards, inclusion in this publication does not constitute a guarantee or endorsement of the quality or value of such product or of the claims made of it by its manufacturer.

Clinics in Sports Medicine (ISSN 0278-5919) is published quarterly by Elsevier Inc., 360 Park Avenue South, New York, NY 10010-1710. Months of issue are January, April, July, and October. Business and Editorial Offices: 1600 John F. Kennedy Blvd., Ste. 1800, Philadelphia, PA 19103-2899. Customer Service Office: 3251 Riverport Lane, Maryland Heights, MO 63043. Periodicals postage paid at New York, NY and additional mailing offices. Subscription prices are $340.00 per year (US individuals), $540.00 per year (US institutions), $165.00 per year (US students), $385.00 per year (Canadian individuals), $666.00 per year (Canadian institutions), $235.00 (Canadian students), $470.00 per year (foreign individuals), $666.00 per year (foreign institutions), and $235.00 per year (foreign students). Foreign air speed delivery is included in all *Clinics* subscription prices. All prices are subject to change without notice. **POSTMASTER:** Send address changes to *Clinics in Sports Medicine*, Elsevier Health Sciences Division, Subscription Customer Service, 3251 Riverport Lane, Maryland Heights, MO 63043. Customer Service (orders, claims, online, change of address): Elsevier Health Sciences Division, Subscription Customer Service, 3251 Riverport Lane, Maryland Heights, MO 63043. Tel: 1-800-654-2452 (U.S. and Canada); 314-447-8871 (outside U.S. and Canada). Fax: 314-447-8029. E-mail: journalscustomerservice-usa@elsevier.com (for print support); journalsonlinesupport-usa@elsevier.com (for online support).

Reprints. For copies of 100 or more of articles in this publication, please contact the Commercial Reprints Department, Elsevier Inc., 360 Park Avenue South, New York, NY 10010-1710. Tel.: 212-633-3874; Fax: 212-633-3820; E-mail: reprints@elsevier.com.

Clinics in Sports Medicine is covered in *MEDLINE/PubMed (Index Medicus) Current Contents/Clinical Medicine, Excerpta Medica,* and *ISI/Biomed.*

Contributors

CONSULTING EDITOR

MARK D. MILLER, MD
Colonel, USAF (Ret), University of Virginia, James Madison University, Charlottesville, Virginia

EDITOR

LTC BRETT D. OWENS, MD, MC, US ARMY
Professor, Uniformed Services University; John A. Feagin Jr. Sports Medicine Fellowship; Orthopaedic Surgery Service, Chief, Department of Orthopaedic Surgery, Keller Army Community Hospital, United States Military Academy, West Point, New York

AUTHORS

ANTHONY I. BEUTLER, MD
Consortium for Health and Military Performance, Uniformed Services University of the Health Sciences, Bethesda, Maryland

COL JOHN A. BOJESCUL, MD
Dwight David Eisenhower Army Medical Center, Fort Gordon, Georgia

TRAVIS C. BURNS, MD
Orthopaedic Surgery Service, San Antonio Military Medical Center, Fort Sam Houston, Texas

KENNETH L. CAMERON, PhD, ATC, MPH
Director of Orthopaedic Research; John A. Feagin Jr. Sports Medicine Fellowship, Department of Orthopaedic Surgery, Keller Army Community Hospital, United States Military Academy, West Point, New York

CPT JAY B. COOK, MD, USA MC
Staff Orthopaedic Surgeon, Winn Army Community Hospital, Fort Stewart, Georgia

SARAH DE LA MOTTE, PhD, MPH, ATC
Consortium for Health and Military Performance, Uniformed Services University of the Health Sciences, Bethesda, Maryland

LINDSAY J. DiSTEFANO, PhD, ATC
Department of Kinesiology, University of Connecticut, Storrs, Connecticut

ALEX DONALDSON, PhD
Deputy Director, Australian Centre for Research into Injury in Sport and its Prevention (ACRISP), Federation University Australia, Ballarat, Victoria, Australia

GUILLAUME D. DUMONT, MD
Assistant Professor, Department of Orthopaedic Surgery and Sports Medicine, University of South Carolina School of Medicine, Columbia, South Carolina

CPT JOHN C. DUNN, MD, MC, USA
Department of Orthopaedic Surgery and Rehabilitation, William Beaumont Army Medical Center, El Paso, Texas

BARNETT FRANK, MA, ATC
Human Movement Science Curriculum, Department of Exercise and Sport Science, University of North Carolina, Chapel Hill, North Carolina

PETAR GOLIJANIN, BS
Research Coordinator, Sports Medicine Service, Massachusetts General Hospital, Boston, Massachusetts

F. WINSTON GWATHMEY Jr, MD
Sports Medicine and Hip Arthroscopy, Assistant Professor, Department of Orthopaedic Surgery, University of Virginia Health System, Charlottesville, Virginia

LTC(P) CHAD A. HALEY, MD
Chief, Department of Surgery, Keller Army Community Hospital, West Point, New York

CAPT JEREMY M. JACOBS, MD
Dwight David Eisenhower Army Medical Center, Fort Gordon, Georgia

Col(s) WARREN R. KADRMAS, MD, MC, USAF
Sports Medicine and Hip Arthroscopy, Department of Orthopaedic Surgery, University of Virginia Health System, Charlottesville, Virginia

STEPHEN W. MARSHALL, PhD
Department of Epidemiology, University of North Carolina, Chapel Hill, North Carolina

JUSTIN D. ORR, MD
Residency Program Director and Chief of Orthopaedic Surgery Foot and Ankle Service, William Beaumont Army Medical Center; Assistant Professor, Department of Orthopaedic Surgery, Texas Tech University Health Sciences Center, El Paso, Texas

LTC BRETT D. OWENS, MD, MC, US ARMY
Professor, Uniformed Services University; John A. Feagin, Jr. Sports Medicine Fellowship; Orthopaedic Surgery Service, Chief, Department of Orthopaedic Surgery, Keller Army Community Hospital, United States Military Academy, West Point, New York

DARIN A. PADUA, PhD, ATC
Department of Exercise and Sport Science, University of North Carolina, Chapel Hill, North Carolina

JEANNE C. PATZKOWSKI, MD
Orthopaedic Surgery Service, San Antonio Military Medical Center, Fort Sam Houston, Texas

CPT ADAM PICKETT, MD, MC, USA
Department of Orthopaedics, Walter Reed National Military Medical Center, Bethesda, Maryland

MATTHEW T. PROVENCHER, MD, CDR, MC, USNR
Associate Professor of Surgery; Chief, Sports Medicine Service, Massachusetts General Hospital, Harvard Medical School, Boston, Massachusetts

JUSTIN ROBBINS, MD
Staff Orthopaedic Surgeon, Madigan Army Medical Center, Tacoma, Washington

CDR JOHN-PAUL RUE, MD, MC, USN
Associate Professor of Surgery, Uniformed Services University of the Health Services, Bethesda, Maryland; Department of Orthopaedics and Sports Medicine, Staff Physician, Naval Health Clinic Annapolis, US Naval Academy, Annapolis, Maryland

COL STEVEN J. SVOBODA, MD
Director, John A. Feagin Jr. Sports Medicine Fellowship, Keller Army Community Hospital, New York

COL JOHN M. TOKISH, MD, MC, USAF
Associate Fellowship Director, Steadman Hawkins Clinic of the Carolinas, Greenville, South Carolina

MAJ BRIAN R. WATERMAN, MD, MC, USA
Assistant Professor, Department of Orthopaedic Surgery and Rehabilitation, Texas Tech University Health Sciences Center, El Paso, Texas; Staff Orthopaedic Surgeon, William Beaumont Army Medical Center, El Paso, Texas; Assistant Professor of Surgery, Uniformed Services University of Health Sciences, Bethesda, Maryland

MAJ MICHAEL A. ZACCHILLI, MD
Department of Orthopaedics and Rehabilitation, Womack Army Medical Center, Fort Bragg, North Carolina

Contents

Because of the volume of sports-related musculoskeletal injuries experienced by military service members, the US Department of Defense has begun to implement the sports medicine model of care to improve the access, efficiency, and effectiveness of care for soldiers who experience musculoskeletal injuries related to sports and training. In this article, the burden of musculoskeletal injuries and conditions related to sports and physical fitness training within the military is reviewed, and the application of the sports medicine model to care for these injuries in military service members is described.

Stress fractures of the lower extremities are common among the military population and athletes. Service members are typically at the greatest risk for stress fracture during basic combat training and initial entry-level training, and it may be related to poor indices of entry-level physical fitness. The purpose of this study is to review the epidemiology and incidence of stress fractures and common stress fractures' diagnosis and treatment and to investigate modifiable and nonmodifiable risk factors and injury prevention. In the soldier or athlete who presents with activity-related pain, stress fractures should be given significant consideration during the clinical evaluation.

Musculoskeletal injuries during military and sport-related training are common, costly, and potentially debilitating. There is a need to develop and implement evidence-based injury prevention strategies to reduce the burden of musculoskeletal injury. The lack of attention to implementation issues is a major factor limiting the ability to successfully reduce musculoskeletal injury rates using evidence-based injury prevention programs. This article proposes 7 steps that can be used to facilitate successful design and implementation of evidence-based injury prevention programs within the logical constraints of a real-world setting by identifying implementation barriers and associated solutions.

Osteoarthritis is observed with a much higher incidence in the military than comparable civilian populations. The diagnosis is often made at a younger age in military members. Anterior cruciate ligament (ACL) ruptures are endemic injuries to the young, active military athlete population. Posttraumatic osteoarthritis (PTOA) occurs commonly in the post-ACL-injured knee. Recent efforts by national organizations have brought attention to the unique opportunity to study PTOA in its earliest, molecular stages in knees sustaining traumatic injuries to the ACL. The search for surrogate biomarkers of PTOA in the military population offers opportunity to advance understanding of this significant disease.

Meniscal tears are more commonly reported in active-duty US military service members than in civilian patient populations. This article presents an overview of meniscal tears as they pertain to the active-duty military population, beginning with the anatomy and biomechanics of the meniscus, types of meniscal tears, and indications for repair. The commonly used techniques for meniscal repair and the success rates and complication of each technique are discussed. The most commonly used technique by the senior author is described, as well as the role for meniscal transplant for treating postmeniscectomy patients in the active-duty military population.

Hip injuries occur commonly in the military. Assessment of the patient with hip pain requires a systematic approach incorporating elements of the history, examination, and imaging. Initial conservative treatment should focus on controlling inflammation and optimizing the biomechanics around the pelvis. Surgery may be indicated in refractory cases with documented intra-articular disorders. Correction of the skeletal deformity contributing to secondary hip damage is essential to ensure durable results. Hip arthroscopy has provided new diagnostic and treatment options and has a growing application in the management of hip injuries in the military population.

Chronic lateral ankle instability is a condition frequently encountered by orthopedic surgeons treating highly active patient populations, particularly military service members. Stress testing and ankle magnetic resonance imaging should be considered during the treatment decision-making process. Appropriate nonoperative treatment should be attempted initially; however, surgical management is warranted to prevent untoward long-term sequelae. Proper surgical treatment and subsequent postoperative management are at the discretion of the individual surgeon but must account for the concomitant diseases associated with chronic lateral ankle instability. Low recurrence of lateral instability can be achieved even in high-demand military patient populations with a focused treatment plan.

Chronic exertional compartment syndrome causes leg pain during exercise and resolves at rest. Paresthesia, especially in the distribution of the superficial peroneal nerve, is common. Nonoperative management may not lead to long-term clinical success. This condition is more difficult to treat in the military setting. Operative treatment is reserved for patients whose symptoms are refractory to conservative management. Fascial decompression has not yielded consistent results in a high-demand cohort, with notable rates of symptom recurrence, incomplete return of physical function, and medical discharge.

Shoulder instability is common in the military population. Such factors as young age, male gender, activity level, and unique job characteristics and duties predispose the military population to increased rates of shoulder instability. The initial treatment of shoulder instability has historically been nonoperative; however, in military personnel who have several characteristics predisposing them to recurrent instability, early surgical intervention may be favorable. Appropriate preoperative imaging and understanding of pathologic lesions are necessary to ensure selection of the appropriate surgical technique. Bony reconstruction procedures, such as the Bristow-Latarjet procedure, iliac crest bone graft, or osteochondral allograft transfer to the anterior glenoid, may be necessary.

Acromioclavicular (AC) dislocations occur frequently in the military population. Most are successfully treated nonoperatively. However, military requirements include more demanding use, resulting in an increased failure rate of conservatively managed AC injuries. Surgical management is indicated for injuries that fail nonoperative treatment, high-grade injuries, and in those patients at high risk for failure of conservative management. No surgical technique is clearly superior but anatomic reconstruction is a consistent procedure with good biomechanical support and growing positive clinical data. There is a substantial risk of failure or complication so the surgeon must approach this injury with meticulous attention.

Chad A. Haley and Michael A. Zacchilli

Pectoralis major (PM) tendon tears are relatively rare injuries that most commonly occur in the 20- to 40 year-old male athlete engaged in weight-lifting exercises, such as when performing a bench press. An accurate and timely diagnosis of a PM tear is important because most studies report better outcomes with acute surgical repair. This article describes the anatomy of the PM muscle, injury epidemiology, tear classification, diagnosis including physical examination and imaging, treatment options for both nonoperative and operative management, complications, a review of the literature including military-related studies, and the authors' preferred technique.

Jeanne C. Patzkowski, Brett D. Owens, and Travis C. Burns

Snapping scapula syndrome is a rare condition that presents with symptoms ranging from crepitus to disabling pain in the scapulothoracic articulation. This condition may be more frequent in a military population because of physical fitness standards that require nonphysiologic forces to be applied to the scapulothoracic articulation. Nonoperative therapy is the first-line management. Surgical options include arthroscopic or open scapulothoracic bursectomy with or without partial scapulectomy. After scapulothoracic arthroscopy up to 90% of patients report good/excellent results, up to 90% are able to return to work, and more than 60% return to sports.

CLINICS IN SPORTS MEDICINE

RELATED INTEREST

Orthopedic Clinics of North America, July 2014 (Vol. 45, No. 3)

CLINICS IN SPORTS MEDICINE

FORTHCOMING ISSUES

January 2015
Sports Hand and Wrist Injuries
Jonathan Isaacs, Editor

July 2015
Sports Cardiology
Robert W. Battle, Editor

October 2015
Sports Injuries in the Foot and Ankle
Anish R. Kadakia, Editor

RECENT ISSUES

July 2014
Understanding the Patellofemoral Joint:
From Instability to Arthroplasty
Alexander K. Meininger, Editor

April 2014
Osteochondritis Dissecans: Diagnosis and
Treatment Options for Athletes
Matthew D. Milewski and
Carl W. Nissen, Editors

January 2014
Unicompartmental Knee Arthroplasty
Keith R. Berend and
Stephanie C. Petterson, Editors

October 2013
Shoulder Instability in the Athlete
Stephen S. Thompson, Editor

RELATED INTEREST

Orthopedic Clinics of North America, July 2014, Vol. 45, No. 3

Foreword

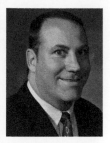

Mark D. Miller, MD
Consulting Editor

Welcome to a special issue of *Clinics in Sports Medicine* featuring military authors and military sports medicine conditions. Of course, a lot of these conditions are not peculiar to the military, so this issue is relevant to all of us that take care of athletes. As a retired military officer myself, I take great pleasure in introducing this issue. The issue is comprehensive, covering both upper and lower extremity conditions. Because of the risk for overuse injuries in this population, this topic is covered extensively. Special thanks to Colonel Brett Owens, who spearheaded this effort as guest editor—it is an outstanding treatise. We dedicate this issue to the coauthor of the last article, Dr Warren Kadrmas. Warren was the victim of a tragic automobile accident recently that unfortunately claimed his life way too early. For those of us that knew him, we all appreciate what a wonderful surgeon, officer, and friend that Dr Kadrmas was. We salute Warren and all that were involved in this special military issue of *Clinics in Sports Medicine*!

Mark D. Miller, MD
University of Virginia
James Madison University
400 Ray C. Hunt Drive, Suite 330
Charlottesville, VA 22908-0159, USA

E-mail address:
MDM3P@hscmail.mcc.virginia.edu

Clin Sports Med 33 (2014) xiii
http://dx.doi.org/10.1016/j.csm.2014.08.001
0278-5919/14/$ – see front matter © 2014 Published by Elsevier Inc.

sportsmed.theclinics.com

Preface

Athletic Injuries in the Military

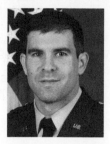

Brett D. Owens, MD, LTC, MC, US ARMY
Editor

Combat is the ultimate contact sport.
—*John A. Feagin Jr, MD*

The subject of this issue of *Clinics in Sports Medicine* is athletic injuries in the military. It has been an honor to have cared for so many fine men and women in uniform over the first decade of my medical career. To be a clinician in the military *is* to practice sports medicine—as athletic injuries are the most common ailments experienced by our fighting forces. This is not intended to slight other fields, but merely to underscore the tremendous burden of disease that musculoskeletal injuries represent. Joint sprains are endemic in the military, with epidemiologic studies showing an incidence rate at an order of magnitude greater than civilian populations. In addition, unique injuries and conditions (uncommon in civilian populations) are often experienced at an appreciably higher rate in the military population due to unique demands placed on the body as part of military training.

The military is an ideal population in which to study athletic injuries, due to the high incidence rates and functional demands, as well as the unique surveillance systems and data available to researchers. This issue boasts authors with varied and robust experience in military orthopedic sports medicine and research and comprises members of all military branches of service, in addition to prominent civilian researchers. Articles detailing injury epidemiology, prevention, and stress fractures are included, in addition to articles focusing on shoulder, hip, knee, and ankle injuries. We hope that this issue has appeal to both military and civilian clinicians and researchers alike, as well as across multiple disciplines. It is my hope that the reader comes away with a

Clin Sports Med 33 (2014) xv–xvi
http://dx.doi.org/10.1016/j.csm.2014.07.001
0278-5919/14/$ – see front matter © 2014 Published by Elsevier Inc.

sportsmed.theclinics.com

greater appreciation for the military service member—as they are truly professional athletes.

Brett D. Owens, MD, LTC, MC, US ARMY
Uniformed Services University
Orthopaedic Surgery
Keller Army Hospital
US Military Academy
West Point, NY 10996, USA

E-mail address:
owensbrett@gmail.com

Dedication

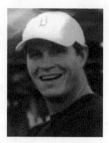

Warren R. Kadrmas, MD, MC, Col(s), USAF

This issue of *Clinics in Sports Medicine* is dedicated to Dr Warren Kadrmas, who trag-ically passed away in April 2014 at the age of 44. Warren was a top military sports sur-geon who was a pioneer in the integration of high-caliber hip arthroscopy as well as cutting-edge shoulder and knee care for our active-duty military personnel. In fact, his article in this issue entitled, "Intra-Articular Hip Pathology in the Military Population: Evaluation and Management," was nearly completed at the time of his untimely pass-ing. It is an honor to have known him over the years, and there is no one who better exemplifies the ideals of a military sports physician.

Warren had spent the majority of his life in the service of the Air Force. He was a distinguished graduate of the US Air Force Academy in 1992, followed by medical school at Duke University, graduating in 1996. He completed both his residency in orthopedic surgery and his fellowship in orthopedic sports medicine at the Hospital for Special Surgery, in New York City. He served the majority of his Air Force career at Wilford Hall Medical Center in San Antonio, Texas. He was routinely recognized for not only his clinical and surgical acumen but also his leadership prowess and held the position of the Orthopaedic Surgery Consultant to the Air Force Surgeon General. In this role, he coordinated all orthopedic assets for the Global War on Terror for the Air Force. He led from the front, serving several tours overseas, often so that others could remain home with family. His quiet self-sacrifice was the hallmark of his leader-ship and inspired a generation of surgeons to serve a mission larger than themselves. He was a prominent researcher and educator and served on numerous peer-review military grant panels as part of the Peer-Reviewed Orthopaedic Research Program. He has been a prominent member of AOSSM and AANA and was in line to be the incoming President of the Society of Military Orthopaedic Surgeons. He was selected for and was scheduled to participate in the AOSSM Traveling Fellowship touring Asia. Warren was one of the finest educators and surgeons we have known and he has touched the lives of countless patients, medical students, and residents, in addition to his fellow clinicians. He is survived by his four beautiful children, Melanie, John Michael, Derek, and Kate; parents, Wayne and Shirley Kadrmas; and brother, Michael Kadrmas, MD.

What we will best remember about Warren is his magnetic personality, charm, wit, and a passion for excellence. Meeting him was making a friend, and working with

Clin Sports Med 33 (2014) xvii–xviii
http://dx.doi.org/10.1016/j.csm.2014.07.002
0278-5919/14/$ – see front matter © 2014 Published by Elsevier Inc.

sportsmed.theclinics.com

him made you want to be better. Warren served with a tireless dedication to the Air Force and was instrumental in advancing the field of military sports surgery. We are lucky to have known him and are humbled by his passing.

Brett D. Owens, MD, LTC, MC, US ARMY
Uniformed Services University
Orthopaedic Surgery
Keller Army Hospital
US Military Academy
West Point, NY 10996, USA

John M. Tokish, MD, COL, MC, USAF
Associate Fellowship Director
Steadman Hawkins Clinic of the Carolinas
200 Patewood C, Suite 100
Greenville, SC 29615, USA

Matthew T. Provencher, MD, CDR, MC, USNR
Sports Medicine Service
Harvard Medical School
Massachusetts General Hospital
175 Cambridge Street, Suite 400
Boston, MA 02114, USA

E-mail address:
owensbrett@gmail.com (B.D. Owens)

The Burden and Management of Sports-Related Musculoskeletal Injuries and Conditions Within the US Military

Kenneth L. Cameron, PhD, MPH, ATC*, Brett D. Owens, MD

KEYWORDS

- Sports medicine • Physical training • Musculoskeletal conditions • Injuries • Military

KEY POINTS

- Musculoskeletal injuries place a significant burden on military service members and the military health system, and they are a leading cause of disability discharge.
- Musculoskeletal injuries and conditions related to sports and physical training account for much lost duty time for military service members and they negatively affect force readiness.
- A leading reason for medical evacuation as a result of nonbattle injuries in soldiers deployed in support of Operation Iraqi Freedom and Operation Enduring Freedom (Afghanistan) was injury related to sports and physical training.
- The types of musculoskeletal injuries and conditions experienced by military service members are consistent with those that are commonly seen in athletic populations and treated in sports medicine clinics.
- Recently, the US Marine Corps, Navy, and Army have recognized the value of the sports medicine model of care to improve the access, efficiency, and effectiveness of care for solders who experience musculoskeletal injuries related to sports and training.

INTRODUCTION

US military service members on active duty comprise a large, predominantly young, and physically active population. According to data from 2011,[1] there were just more than 1.4 million military personnel on active duty, most of whom were men (85.5%) and enlisted soldiers, with a ratio of 5 enlisted soldiers for every officer. Half

Disclosure: The authors are employees of the federal government and the views and opinions expressed in this manuscript are those of the authors and do not reflect the views or official policies of the Department of the Army, The Department of Defense, or the U.S. Government.
Department of Orthopaedic Surgery, Keller Army Hospital, United States Military Academy, 900 Washington Road, West Point, NY 10996, USA
* Corresponding author.
E-mail address: kenneth.l.cameron.civ@mail.mil

Clin Sports Med 33 (2014) 573–589
http://dx.doi.org/10.1016/j.csm.2014.06.004
0278-5919/14/$ – see front matter Published by Elsevier Inc.

sportsmed.theclinics.com

of the approximately 1.2 million enlisted soldiers are 25 years of age or younger and more than 70% are 30 years of age or younger.[1] Musculoskeletal injuries are endemic within the military population, and they pose the greatest public health problem facing military service members during both peacetime and combat operations. Musculo-skeletal injuries and conditions are also the greatest threat to military readiness.[2] Research in civilian populations has shown that individuals younger than 30 years are at increased risk for several sports-related musculoskeletal injuries and condi-tions.[3] Considering the demographic composition of the US military population, it is not surprising that sports-related musculoskeletal injuries and conditions are perva-sive within the ranks.

Many of the musculoskeletal injuries and conditions experienced by US military service members are related to participation in sports, recreation, and physical training.[4–8] As a result, military service members are at substantially increased risk for musculoskeletal injuries and conditions that are commonly seen in athletes and managed in sports medicine clinics, when compared with the general population.[9] Athletic injuries are also the leading cause of disability discharge among military ser-vice members in the US Army, according to Physical Evaluation Board data.[10] In this article, the burden of musculoskeletal injuries and conditions within the military related to sports and physical fitness training is reviewed, and how the sports medicine model (eg, bringing medical resources with specialized training in musculoskeletal injuries to the training environment) is being applied to care for these injuries in military service members is described.

MUSCULOSKELETAL INJURIES RELATED TO SPORTS AND PHYSICAL TRAINING

Musculoskeletal injuries and conditions related to sports and physical training account for much lost duty time among military service members, and they negatively affect force readiness.[4] Lauder and colleagues[4] examined hospitalizations as a result of injuries related to sport and physical training in US Army personnel on active duty between 1989 and 1994. Most of these injuries affected the lower extremity, with the knee being the most common site of injury, followed by the ankle, heel and foot, and lower leg. The hand, shoulder, forearm, and wrist were the most common sites of injury in the upper extremity. Bone fractures (33%) were the most common type of injury associated with sports and physical training, followed by sprains and strains (29%), joint dislocations (15%), and concussions (5%). The most common activities associated with injury were basketball, football, softball, and physical fitness training in men, whereas physical fitness training was the most common activity associated with injury in women, followed by basketball, softball, and skiing.

In a series of recent studies, Burnham and colleagues[5–8] reviewed safety data within the US Air Force to examine the most common events that produce injury resulting in lost duty time over a 10-year period between 1993 and 2002. Sports-related injuries were second only to motor vehicle–related injuries in the total number of injuries reported and the total days lost from duty as a result of injury. Although fewer than 16% of motor vehicle–related injuries occurred on base, more than 70% of all sports-related injuries occurred on military installations.[8] Similar to the results reported by Lauder and colleagues[4] for hospitalizations, basketball, softball, and flag football, respectively, were the most common sports-related activities that resulted in time loss injuries among service members.[8] Average time loss because of sports-related injuries was 6 days (median = 2–3 days), regardless of whether airmen were injured in basketball, softball, or football. Injuries resulting from basketball were most commonly the result of jumping or landing awkwardly (26%), jumping and landing on another player's foot (17%), or colliding with another player (10%).[5] The most common types of injuries reported as a result of playing basketball were sprains (38%), followed by fractures (24%), strains (15%), and tendon ruptures (11%).[5] Injuries resulting from softball were most commonly the result of sliding (23%), being hit by a bat (20%), colliding with another player (16%), or running (11%).[7] Approximately two-thirds of all injuries as a result of softball were fractures, sprains, and strains; however, fractures accounted for 40% of all injuries and were the most common injury regardless of mechanism.[7] Injuries resulting from participation in flag football most frequently resulted from contact with another player (42%), slipping, tripping, or falling (14%), running and sprinting (11%), and planting, cutting, and changing direction (7%).[6] The most common types of injuries reported as a result of playing flag football were fractures (36%), sprains and strains (34%), and joint dislocations (7%).[6] The findings of these studies further suggest that military service members experience a significant number of sports-related musculoskeletal injuries and that these injuries result in considerable time loss, which affects force readiness. The findings also suggest that more than 70% of sports-related injuries occur on military installations, where military leaders may play a direct role in implementing and enforcing policies that can mitigate the risk of injury caused by sports participation among military service members.

In addition to organized and unorganized athletics, military service members frequently participate in physical fitness training, and injuries as a result of physical training are common.[11–13] Affectionately referred to as PT (physical training), or most recently PRT (physical readiness training), these mandatory sessions are typically conducted 3 to 5 times per week for about an hour and consist of running, muscular strength and endurance training, speed and agility training, or calisthenics. Lauder and colleagues[4] also detailed the burden of PT-related injuries and found that this activity was eclipsed only by basketball, football, and softball for injuries in men. In women, physical training was the activity resulting in most injuries. Similar to the other sporting activities, approximately 40% of injuries are confined to the ankle and knee.[4] Because the US Army has recently encouraged combatives training during unit PT time, an increase in upper extremity sprains has been noted by some providers.[14] Recently, the prevention of musculoskeletal injuries related to sports and physical training has been identified as a top priority for injury prevention across the Department of Defense.[15,16]

DEPLOYMENT-RELATED MUSCULOSKELETAL INJURIES AND CONDITIONS

Krentz and colleagues[17] reported that sports injuries are also a significant threat to force readiness among US Navy personnel deployed on an aircraft carrier. These investigators examined injuries among naval personnel aboard the USS *Theodore Roosevelt*, a nuclear-powered aircraft carrier with 5800 sailors aboard, during a 6-month deployment. Participation in sports and recreational activities resulted in 19% of all injuries and 25% of injuries that led to lost duty time. Most injuries documented were musculoskeletal injuries that affected the lower extremity. Basketball resulted in most musculoskeletal injuries that were associated with lost duty time, followed by volleyball, football, and weight lifting. The most common types of injuries documented were sprains and fractures. The investigators noted that injury prevention strategies that target high-risk sports and recreational activities might substantially mitigate the burden of these musculoskeletal injuries during deployment aboard aircraft carriers and similar vessels and might limit the associated impact on force readiness.[17]

Despite the volume of news reports focused on battle-related injuries resulting from the recent conflicts in Iraq and Afghanistan, soldiers were 2 to 4 times as likely to be medically evacuated from the war zone as a result of nonbattle injuries, according to a study by Hauret and colleagues.[18] The number 1 reason for medical evacuation as a result of nonbattle injuries in soldiers deployed in support of Operation Iraqi Freedom and Operation Enduring Freedom (Afghanistan) was injury related to sports and physical training.[18] Previous military operations, for which comparable data are available (Desert Shield and Desert Storm), also suggest that injury related to sports and physical training was among the top reasons for medical evacuation for nonbattle injuries.[19] More than 80% of the nonbattle injuries examined by Hauret and colleagues[18] that resulted in medical evacuation were classified as acute traumatic injuries or injury-related musculoskeletal conditions. The most common musculoskeletal injuries and conditions that resulted in medical evacuation because of nonbattle injury included fractures, inflammation and pain caused by overuse injury, joint dislocations, sprains and strains, and internal joint derangement (eg, meniscus tears, anterior cruciate ligament [ACL] rupture, articular cartilage lesions). The most common anatomic sites of nonbattle injury requiring medical evacuation included the back, knee, wrist and hand, ankle and foot, and shoulder, respectively. Belmont and colleagues[20] reported similar findings for diagnoses and anatomic site of nonbattle musculoskeletal injuries among a US Army Brigade Combat Team deployed during Operation Iraqi Freedom. These data indicate that more military service members are medically evacuated from theater for nonbattle injuries, and injuries related to sports and physical training are the leading cause of nonbattle injuries, significant enough to require medical evacuation among deployed soldiers. The data also suggest that musculoskeletal injuries commonly seen in sports medicine clinics likely have the greatest impact on force readiness, even during times of war.

In addition to the burden of nonbattle injuries significant enough to require medical evacuation from theater, many soldiers returning from a full combat deployment present with nonemergent musculoskeletal injuries and conditions that require medical care.[21] These injuries may be disregarded as insignificant in the combat environment, may be ignored by soldiers wanting to stay with their unit and fellow soldiers, or may be identified as insufficient to warrant medical evacuation when service members are treated in theater and returned to duty.[21] Goodman and colleagues[21] examined these nonemergent musculoskeletal injuries and conditions in a US Army Brigade Combat Team returning from a 15-month deployment in support of Operation Iraqi Freedom. A total of 731 orthopedic consultations were conducted among the 3787 soldiers who completed the deployment without being medically evacuated. Nearly 90% of the injuries or conditions warranting consultation were the result of nonbattle musculoskeletal injuries or exacerbation of a previous injury or condition during deployment. Four percent of the soldiers (n=140) returning from deployment required an orthopedic surgical procedure as a result of their injury. Although the investigators were unable to systematically document the cause of injury in these service members, it is reasonable to assume that many of these injuries and conditions were likely caused by sports participation and physical training, based on the available epidemiologic data.[18] Furthermore, the types of procedures performed in these returning service members are consistent with those that would be performed in an orthopedic sports medicine clinic or service. The most frequently performed procedures were to treat internal derangement of the knee (eg, meniscus tears, ACL rupture, articular cartilage lesions), shoulder instability (eg, dislocations and subluxations), and superior labrum anterior to posterior (SLAP) lesions.[21] These injuries included 19 first-time anterior shoulder dislocations/subluxations and 18 ACL ruptures. Although there were few similar studies for the investigators to compare their results, they suggest that the spectrum of musculoskeletal injuries and conditions seen in these service members after a full combat deployment most closely approximate those commonly reported among elite athletes.[21]

MUSCULOSKELETAL INJURIES AND CONDITIONS COMMONLY SEEN IN SPORTS MEDICINE CLINICS

In recent years, investigators have begun to examine the burden of many musculoskeletal injuries and conditions, which are commonly seen in athletic populations and sports medicine clinics, within the active duty military population. This research has included a series of population-based epidemiologic studies using data from the Defense Medical Surveillance System and other databases to systematically evaluate the burden of musculoskeletal injuries and conditions affecting military service members.[22–40] These studies initially focused on acute traumatic joint injuries that typically lead to significant time loss from duty, increased morbidity, and the need for surgical intervention. These reports documented the incidence rates of several specific musculoskeletal injuries among military service members on active duty. The reports also examined the demographic and occupational risk factors associated with these conditions. These data have been critical in defining the scope of the injury problem within the military, identifying the groups at highest risk for certain injuries, and have been helpful in targeting high-risk populations for injury prevention interventions. This section provides an overview of the important findings from these studies.

Injuries to the Knee

Owens and colleagues[33] examined the incidence of ACL injuries among military personnel on active duty over a 7-year period from 1997 to 2003 inclusive. These investigators observed that the incidence rate of ACL injury among military service members on active duty was more than 10 times higher when compared with previously published rates within the general population.[33] The investigators also observed that men experience significantly higher incidence rates for ACL injury when compared with female service members. This finding may reflect differences in occupational physical tasks and activities between men and women serving in the military, because previous studies have reported that women are at greater risk to ACL injury when compared with men engaging in similar high-risk activities, controlling for athletic exposure (eg, basketball).[41]

Jones and colleagues[36] conducted a similar study examining the incidence rate of meniscus tear in the knee among military service members on active duty. Similar to the results for ACL injury, the incidence of meniscus tears was more than 10 times higher among military service members compared with previous reports in the general population, and the rate for men was nearly 20% higher compared with women. Injuries affected the medial meniscus twice as frequently as the lateral meniscus, which is similar to previous reports. The investigators also observed that increased age was associated with the increased incidence of acute meniscus tears within the military population on active duty after controlling for other potentially confounding variables (**Fig. 1**). Occupational factors, including rank and branch of military service, were also associated with the incidence of meniscus tears, with those in the Army and Marine Corps and serving in the enlisted ranks experiencing the highest rates of injury.

Hsiao and colleagues[35] examined the incidence rate of patellar dislocation within the military population on active duty. These investigators reported that the incidence rate for patellar dislocation was again nearly 10 times higher within the military

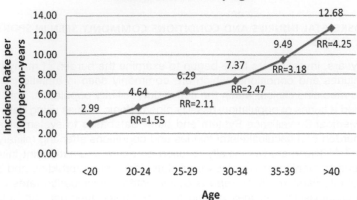

Fig. 1. Adjusted incidence rates and rate ratios for meniscal injuries among all active duty US service members by age between 1998 and 2006. Adjusted for sex, race, branch of military service, and military rank. Age younger than 20 years used as referent category. RR, incidence rate ratio. (*From* Jones JC, Burks R, Owens BD, et al. Incidence and risk factors associated with meniscal injuries among active-duty US Military Service Members. J Athl Train 2012;47(1):70; with permission.)

population on active duty compared with other estimates from the general population[42,43]; however, their findings were similar to a previous study examining the incidence of patellar dislocation in the Finnish military.[44] This study was the first population-based study with adequate power to examine differences in the incidence rate for patellar dislocation between men and women. The incidence rate among women was 61% higher when compared with men after controlling for age, race, branch of military service, and military rank. Contrary to the findings for meniscus tears, the risk of patellar dislocation decreased with increasing age. Consistent with the other studies, service in the Army and Marine Corps and enlisted ranks was associated with higher incidence rates of patellar dislocation.

Similar studies have reported the significance of ACL injuries within the military. According to Lauder and colleagues,[4] ACL injuries were the leading cause of hospitalizations in the US Army because of injury related to sports and physical training. Nearly 10% of military service members who sustain an ACL injury are discharged from military service because of disability as a direct result of the injury,[45] and those who elect conservative management rather than surgical reconstruction are at increased risk for reinjury, subsequent surgery, and disability discharge.[46] It is also likely that up to 50% go on to experience degenerative joint changes after ACL injury, which may contribute to the rapid progression of posttraumatic osteoarthritis (OA).[47,48] This situation can lead to disability discharge, and degenerative arthritis is a leading cause of disability in military populations.[10] Lauder and colleagues[4] also reported that meniscus injuries were second only to ACL injuries for sports-related hospitalizations among service members in the US Army. The long-term burden of meniscus injuries is also significant, because these have been associated with a high incidence and the rapid progression of posttraumatic OA.[47,49] In a recent study, sports-related knee injuries were also reported to cause a significant burden in terms of hospitalization, surgery, and long-term disability in the Finnish military.[50]

Injuries to the Ankle

Ankle sprain injuries are common among US military service members, and these injuries typically result in significant time loss and persistent disability.[51] Furthermore, ankle sprain injuries are second only to low back pain in relation to the overall percentage of the rehabilitation workload in military populations.[52] Cameron and colleagues[30] conducted a population-based retrospective cohort study to examine the incidence rate of ankle sprain injuries in active duty military personnel, using similar methods and data from the Defense Medical Surveillance System. The incidence rate for ankle sprain injuries within the active duty military population was notably higher (5–6.6 times) compared with studies performed in the general population.[53] Women experienced higher incidence rates for ankle sprain compared with men in all branches of military service, except the US Air Force, in which there was no difference between men and women. Again, men and women serving in the Army and Marine Corps experienced the highest incidence rates for ankle sprain injuries (**Fig. 2**). As a result, it is not surprising that chronic ankle instability associated with ankle sprain is common within military populations.

Injuries to the Shoulder

Military service members on active duty have significant upper extremity occupational demands and physical training requirements. As a result, injuries to the shoulder, such

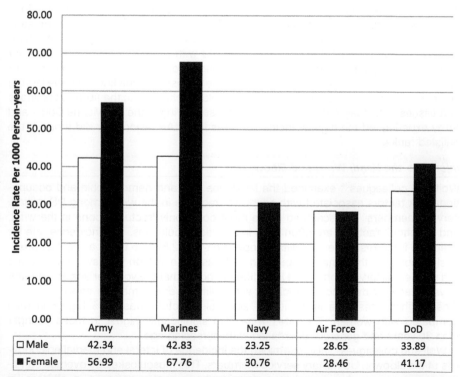

	Army	Marines	Navy	Air Force	DoD
☐ Male	42.34	42.83	23.25	28.65	33.89
■ Female	56.99	67.76	30.76	28.46	41.17

Fig. 2. Incidence of ankle sprains by service and sex in the US military. DoD, Department of Defense. (*From* Cameron KL, Owens BD, DeBerardino TM. Incidence of ankle sprains among active duty members of the United States Armed Services between 1998-2006. J Athl Train 2010;45(1):32; with permission.)

as glenohumeral joint dislocation, are common and often require surgical repair. Owens and colleagues[32] conducted a population-based study using data extracted from the Defense Medical Surveillance System to examine the incidence of shoulder dislocation injuries in this population. A secondary objective was to identify occupational and demographic factors associated with shoulder dislocation injuries. The investigators reported that the incidence rate for shoulder dislocation injuries in the US military population was 7 to 21 times higher compared with previous studies and published estimates in the general population.[54] However, the rate was not as high as that observed in military cadets in a separate study.[55] Furthermore, the incidence rate for men was nearly twice as high compared with women. Those in the age group younger than 20 years experienced the highest incidence rate of injury, and the risk of injury decreased with increasing age. Again, those serving in the US Army and Marine Corps and in the enlisted ranks experienced the highest incidence rates for shoulder dislocation. Similar to the rates associated with ACL injuries, data suggest that approximately 9% of service members on active duty who require Bankart repair after shoulder instability are discharged for disability because of their injury.[56]

Waterman and colleagues[57] recently examined trends in the incidence rate of physician-diagnosed SLAP lesions in the shoulder within the military population on active duty. These investigators reported that the overall incidence rate for SLAP lesions in this population was 2.13 per 1000 person-years during the 8-year study period and that there was a significant 21.2% annual increase in the incidence rate over time. There was also a significant association between age and the incidence rate for SLAP lesions within this population. On average, there was a 24.5% increase in the incidence rate for SLAP lesions with every 5 years of advancing age after controlling for important confounding variables. As with meniscus injuries, the risk for SLAP lesion injuries increased with increasing age. This is likely because age-related degeneration has been noted in both the meniscus in the knee and the labrum in the shoulder, which occurs because of histologic changes in the fibrocartilaginous soft tissues.[58] Similar to the other studies, those serving in the US Marine Corps and Army experienced the highest incidence rates for SLAP lesions, as did those in the enlisted ranks.

Injuries to the Hand, Wrist, and Elbow

Wolf and colleagues[24] examined the incidence rate and demographic and occupational risk factors associated with scaphoid fractures in the wrist among US military service members. The scaphoid is the most commonly fractured bone in the wrist, and scaphoid fractures are often seen in athletic populations. The incidence rate for scaphoid fractures in the US military population was 2.5 to 15 times as high as previously reported in the general population and was twice as high as previously reported in a smaller military cohort.[24] The investigators noted that the younger age and greater physical activity demands associated with military service may be associated with these higher rates. The incidence of scaphoid fracture was 55% higher in men compared with women. The rates were also significantly higher in those younger than 30 years and generally decreased with increasing age.

Wolf and colleagues[34] also examined the incidence of lateral and medial epicondylitis of the elbow in US military service members. This musculoskeletal overuse condition, more commonly referred to as tennis elbow, is also common in athletes. In military service members, the incidence rate of lateral epicondylitis was 22% higher compared with men, but there was no difference between men and women for medial epicondylitis. Increasing age was associated with an increased risk of both medial and lateral epicondylitis; however, the magnitude of the increase in risk was larger for the latter. The incidence rate of lateral epicondylitis was 4 times as high as the rate for medial epicondylitis in military service members.

Other Overuse Injuries and Chronic Conditions

Although acute traumatic injuries are common in the military, overuse injuries affecting the musculoskeletal system are also a significant concern, particularly during initial entry level training on joining the military. Many of the overuse injuries that are common in military service members are also common in athletes. Stress fracture injuries are a debilitating condition associated with several weight-bearing sports and physical activities, and these injuries are also pervasive in military training populations.[59] Knapik and colleagues[59] recently examined the demographic and physical risk factors associated with stress fracture in a large cohort of US Army personnel going through basic training. These investigators reported that older age, lower body weight, lower body mass index, and race/ethnicity other than black were associated with increased rates of stress fracture, regardless of sex. When examining men only, increased height and weight were also associated with the increased risk of stress fracture during basic combat training. The investigators also observed that the incidence of stress fracture among women was approximately 4 to 5 times higher compared with men, which has consistently been reported in many previous studies. A more detailed examination of stress fractures within military populations is provided by Bojescul and colleagues elsewhere in this issue.

Lower extremity tendinopathies are common in athletes, as well as in US military service members. Scher and colleagues[28] examined the incidence rate of plantar fasciitis within military service members on active duty. These investigators reported an overall incidence rate of 10.5 cases per 1000 person-years. The incidence rate among women was significantly higher, nearly twice as high, compared with men. Incidence rates were highest in those service members who were younger than 20 years and those who were older than 40 years. After controlling for other potential confounding factors, senior officers were at the greatest risk for being diagnosed with plantar fasciitis. Owens and colleagues[60] examined the incidence and risk factors associated with lower extremity tendinopathies within the Millennium Cohort of military service members. Specifically, these investigators examined rates and risk factors for Achilles tendinopathy, patellar tendinopathy, and plantar fasciitis in military service members on active duty enrolled in the parent cohort study. Service members who were overweight, and those who reported moderate weekly alcohol consumption at baseline, were at significantly higher risk for Achilles tendinopathy, and the risk of Achilles tendinopathy increased with increasing age.[60] Those serving in the army were at significantly higher risk compared with those serving in the US Navy and Air Force. Service members with a history of Achilles tendinopathy were more than 3 times as likely to develop subsequent tendinopathy. In contrast to the findings for Achilles tendinopathy, younger service members experienced higher rates of patellar tendinopathy, and the rate generally decreased with increasing age. Again, those serving in the army were at the greatest risk for patellar tendinopathy, and those with a history of previous tendinopathy at baseline were more than 3 times as likely to experience patellar tendinopathy during follow-up. Service members who had recently deployed at baseline were more likely to be diagnosed with plantar fasciitis during follow-up. Individuals who were overweight at baseline were also at greater risk for being diagnosed with plantar fasciitis, similar to those with Achilles tendinopathy. As observed for the other tendinopathies, those serving in the army were at increased risk for plantar fasciitis during follow-up. As reported previously by Scher and colleagues,[28] women and increasing age were also associated with the increased incidence of plantar fasciitis during follow-up in the Millennium Cohort.

Degenerative Joint Disease in Military Populations

There is substantial evidence, in both animal and human studies, to support the link between traumatic joint injury and the subsequent occurrence of degenerative joint disease and OA. Because of the higher rates of joint injury observed among military populations and the significant demands of occupational and physical training in this population, similar epidemiologic studies[23] were conducted using data from the Defense Medical Surveillance System to examine the incidence rate and burden of OA among military service members. The investigators hypothesized that the rates of degenerative joint disease in military personnel on active duty would be significantly higher compared with the general population. The investigators observed that the incidence rate for OA was significantly higher in every age group of military service members compared with the general population, and the disparity between military service members and the general population increased with increasing age (**Fig. 3**). Although the investigators were unable to link the increased incidence rate of OA in this study to a history of previous joint injury, they speculated that the increased incidence rates observed in the military population were likely a function of the high rates of joint injury and the cumulative stress associated with the physical demands associated with years of military service.

In a separate study, Scher and colleagues[27] examined the incidence of hip OA among military service members on active duty. The overall incidence rate for men

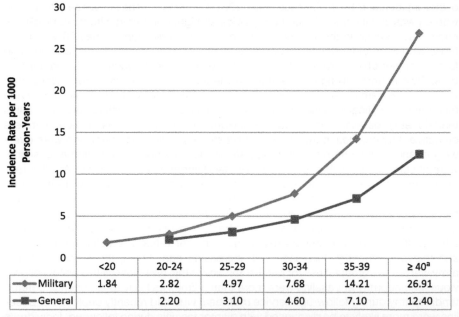

	<20	20-24	25-29	30-34	35-39	≥ 40[a]
Military	1.84	2.82	4.97	7.68	14.21	26.91
General		2.20	3.10	4.60	7.10	12.40

Fig. 3. Comparison of unadjusted incidence rates for OA between military and general populations by age. [a] Incidence rate data for the 40 to 44 and 45 to 49 year groups were combined for this category in the general population. (*From* Cameron KL, Hsiao MS, Owens BD, et al. Incidence of physician-diagnosed osteoarthritis among active duty United States military service members. Arthritis Rheum 2011;63(10):2978; with permission.)

was 35 cases per 100,000 person-years, with rates ranging from 32 cases per 100,000 person-years in men to 54 cases per 100,000 person-years in women. Although these investigators observed lower incidence rates for hip OA than previously reported in the literature, this is likely because most published studies have focused on the incidence of OA in older study populations. The observed incidence rates for hip OA in this relatively young and healthy population are disconcerting, and combined with the overall rates for OA compared with the general population, raise concerns about the burden of OA in load-bearing joints after years of military service.

This section highlights a series of studies that have examined the incidence and burden of musculoskeletal injuries and conditions within the US military population on active duty. These studies provide a perspective on the spectrum and impact of musculoskeletal injuries and conditions experienced by US military service members on active duty. The studies also provide insight into the demographic and occupational risk factors within this population. In general, acute traumatic joint injuries and fractures seem to be more common in younger service members, and the risk of these injuries decreases with increasing age. Conversely, the risk for chronic overuse injuries, injuries to the fibrocartilage in the knee and shoulder, and degenerative joint disease and OA is lowest in younger age groups and increases with increasing age. There are also clear gender influences on injury risk within the US military population. Those serving in the US Army and Marine Corps, and those in the junior and senior enlisted ranks, are at the greatest risk for several musculoskeletal injuries and conditions, as documented in this section. These data can be helpful in planning and targeting potential injury prevention initiatives within this high-risk population.

APPLYING THE SPORTS MEDICINE MODEL IN THE MILITARY SETTING

Because of the large volume and type of musculoskeletal injuries commonly experienced by US military service members, the sports medicine model of care, which has traditionally been used to treat elite athletes, offers many potential advantages associated with access to services and the delivery of medical care in this population. The sports medicine model brings medical assets to the training environment, in which most musculoskeletal injuries occur. Traditionally, this environment has been the sideline during athletic practices and competitions. This model facilitates the rapid initial assessment and management of injuries, with the major goals of mitigating the secondary effects of injury and returning athletes to participation as quickly and safely as possible. The sports medicine model also uses a team approach, in which allied health care providers, typically athletic trainers, initially evaluate and triage injured athletes and coordinate care, making rapid referrals to appropriate providers and allied health care professionals for follow-up evaluation and care as needed. Because athletic trainers possess expertise in musculoskeletal injuries related to sports and training, fewer nonsurgical patients are typically referred for specialty care (eg, orthopedic surgery), unless such care is indicated. Also, more patients can typically be seen in a shorter time in a traditional open-bay training room–style clinical environment. This model typically allows the multidisciplinary team of health care providers to see patients simultaneously during designated clinic hours and consult with one another on diagnoses and treatment plans, which is efficient for the patient. The sports medicine model of care is equally focused on primary injury prevention, because primary prevention is the best way to keep athletes on the field and in the game. This focus is of primary importance within the military setting, to optimize force readiness.

Conversely, the traditional medical model used throughout the military health system requires patients to schedule an appointment, typically with a primary care provider, who initially assesses the nature of the injury and serves as the gatekeeper to additional services. Often, these primary care providers have limited training in the treatment and management of musculoskeletal injuries, which may result in referral to physical therapy or orthopedic surgery for further evaluation and management, requiring additional appointments and further delays in care and suboptimal treatment outcomes for an injury.[61] Such delays may have significant consequences for service members on active duty, resulting in failure to complete training requirements, missed deployments, and decreased readiness in operational units.[61]

Recognizing the value-added benefits of the sports medicine model in a military training environment, the US military has recently shown significant interest in implementing and expanding this approach to health care delivery. The US Marine Corps and the US Navy have led the way in establishing the military sports medicine model and deploying highly skilled allied health care professionals with specialty training in musculoskeletal injury assessment and management to military training sites. Although the benefits of the sports medicine model were discussed in the 1990s, it was not until the turn of the century that the concept gained traction. Recognizing the cost of training-related musculoskeletal injuries, in 2002 the US Marine Corps developed and initially piloted the 27-month Sports Medicine and Injury Prevention (SMIP) initiative.[62] The main objective of the SMIP was the primary prevention of musculoskeletal injuries; however, it was expected that secondary and tertiary prevention benefits would also be realized from the initiative.[62] The initiative stood up training room facilities and embedded athletic trainers in the field environment at key training sites, typically at the battalion aid station level, at 6 Marine Corps training sites. The initial results of the SMIP were promising and resulted in the expansion of the program to other training sites and within special operations units. The Marine Corps is looking to expand this program and provide sports medicine and athletic training support at the company level within some infantry units.

In coordination with the implementation of the SMIP, the US Navy committed to establishing and operating Sports Medicine and Rehabilitation Team (SMART) clinics at the 6 training sites identified for the SMIP pilot project.[62] Although the SMART clinics were run and staffed by the military treatment facility (MTF) responsible for providing medical care at each training site, the clinics were located in the training area rather than the MTF, facilitating better access for soldiers. The original staffing plan for the SMART clinics was to include a primary care sports medicine physician, a physical therapist, and athletic trainers. Although limited data are available on the optimal staffing of these military sports medicine facilities, Masters[62] reported that staffing SMART clinics with a primary care sports medicine physician, a physical therapist, 2 athletic trainers, 2 corpsman, and an administrative assistant permitted the facility to see approximately 1000 patients per month and presented the best business case analysis for the facility. Like the SMIP program, the SMART clinic model has expanded significantly within the Navy medicine footprint over the past 10 years since it was initially implemented at military training sites. In one of the few published reports on the model, Brawley and colleagues[61] recently reported that the SMART clinic model resulted in a 9% to 31% relative reduction in orthopedic consults, a 40% relative reduction in Physical Evaluation Board (eg, review for medical discharge) referrals among those with time loss injuries, and an increase in patient encounters, suggesting increased efficiency and access to care and mitigating losses because of injury.

Based on the success of the sports medicine model implemented by the Marine Corps and Navy, and preliminary pilot projects at Fort Jackson, South Carolina and Fort Campbell, Kentucky, the US Army Medical Command and the US Army Training and Doctrine Command collaborated to develop and pilot musculoskeletal action teams (MATs). Similar to the goals of the SMIP and SMART clinic initiatives, the MATs use the sports medicine model and focus on 3 primary principles: (1) injury prevention, (2) precision in executing physical readiness training, and (3) optimizing human performance.[63] The MATs are assigned at the brigade level and include 2 physical therapists, 2 physical therapy technicians, 4 athletic trainers, and 4 strength and conditioning coaches. Unlike the SMART clinics, the MATs are led not by a primary care sports medicine physician but by a physical therapist. The initial 2-year MAT pilot project was initiated at 6 army training sites, including Fort Benning, Fort Lee, Fort Sill, Fort Jackson, and Fort Leonard Wood, in April, 2011 and concluded in April, 2013. The primary outcome metrics evaluated during this pilot project were related to fitness indices, injury rates, and attrition during training. Although the results of this pilot project have not been published or widely disseminated, in July, 2013, Fort Benning issued a contract solicitation to provide athletic training and strength and conditioning services in support of the MAT program,[64] and continuation of the initial pilot initiative was supported to some degree at all sites that initially implemented the MAT program. At a minimum, this observation indicates that the program was viewed as a success in the eyes of the local command(s) where this model was implemented.

SUMMARY

Military service members comprise a young and physically active population who are at increased risk for musculoskeletal injuries and conditions related to sports and physical training. Even during times of war, musculoskeletal injuries and conditions related to sports and physical training, not associated with combat, are the leading cause of medical evacuation from theater. As a result, these injuries significantly compromise military readiness, and they can lead to an increased risk for reinjury and long-term disability among military service members. Regardless of the mechanism of injury, the large volume and types of musculoskeletal injuries and conditions that affect soldiers are similar to those that are commonly seen and treated in sports medicine clinics and practices. Recently, the US Marine Corps, Navy, and Army have recognized the value of the sports medicine model of care to improve the access, efficiency, and effectiveness of care for solders who experience musculoskeletal injuries related to sports and training. A highly skilled sports medicine team of providers and allied health care professionals (eg, athletic trainers, physical therapists), with expertise in the prevention, assessment, diagnosis, and management of musculoskeletal injuries and conditions, will continue to be an integral cog in the effective management of these types of injuries into the future, as the sports medicine model continues to expand across the military health system.

REFERENCES

1. Office of the Deputy Under Secretary of Defense for Military Community and Family Policy. 2011 demographics: profile of the military community. Arlington (VA): Department of Defense; 2012. p. 217.
2. Jones BH, Canham-Chervak M, Sleet DA. An evidence-based public health approach to injury priorities and prevention recommendations for the U.S. Military. Am J Prev Med 2010;38(Suppl 1):S1–10.
3. Gotsch K, Annest JL, Holmgreen P, et al. Nonfatal sports- and recreation-related injuries treated in emergency departments–United States, July 2000–June 2001. MMWR Morb Mortal Wkly Rep 2002;51(33):736–40.
4. Lauder TD, Baker SP, Smith GS, et al. Sports and physical training injury hospitalizations in the army. Am J Prev Med 2000;18(3 Suppl):118–28.

5. Burnham BR, Copley GB, Shim MJ, et al. Mechanisms of basketball injuries reported to the HQ Air Force Safety Center a 10-year descriptive study, 1993-2002. Am J Prev Med 2010;38(1 Suppl):S134–40.

6. Burnham BR, Copley GB, Shim MJ, et al. Mechanisms of flag-football injuries reported to the HQ Air Force Safety Center a 10-year descriptive study, 1993-2002. Am J Prev Med 2010;38(1 Suppl):S141–7.

7. Burnham BR, Copley GB, Shim MJ, et al. Mechanisms of slow-pitch softball injuries reported to the HQ Air Force Safety Center a 10-year descriptive study, 1993-2002. Am J Prev Med 2010;38(1 Suppl):S126–33.

8. Copley GB, Burnham BR, Shim MJ, et al. Using safety data to describe common injury-producing events examples from the U.S. Air force. Am J Prev Med 2010; 38(1 Suppl):S117–25.

9. Knapik J, Ang P, Reynolds K, et al. Physical fitness, age, and injury incidence in infantry soldiers. J Occup Med 1993;35(6):598–603.

10. Amoroso PJ, Canham ML. Disabilities related to the musculoskeletal system: physical evaluation board data. In: Atlas of injuries in the U.S. Armed Forces. Fort Detrick (MD): US Army Medical Research and Material Command; 1999.

11. Jones BH, Cowan DN, Tomlinson JP, et al. Epidemiology of injuries associated with physical training among young men in the army. Med Sci Sports Exerc 1993;25(2):197–203.

12. Jones BH, Knapik JJ. Physical training and exercise-related injuries. Surveillance, research and injury prevention in military populations. Sports Med 1999;27(2):111–25.

13. Knapik JJ, Sharp MA, Canham-Chervak M, et al. Risk factors for training-related injuries among men and women in basic combat training. Med Sci Sports Exerc 2001;33(6):946–54.

14. Possley DR, Johnson AE. Musculoskeletal injuries sustained in modern army combatives. Mil Med 2012;177(1):60–3.

15. Bullock SH, Jones BH, Gilchrist J, et al. Prevention of physical training-related injuries recommendations for the military and other active populations based on expedited systematic reviews. Am J Prev Med 2010;38(1 Suppl): S156–81.

16. Ruscio BA, Jones BH, Bullock SH, et al. A process to identify military injury prevention priorities based on injury type and limited duty days. Am J Prev Med 2010;38(1 Suppl):S19–33.

17. Krentz MJ, Li G, Baker SP. At work and play in a hazardous environment: injuries aboard a deployed U.S. Navy aircraft carrier. Aviat Space Environ Med 1997; 68(1):51–5.

18. Hauret KG, Taylor BJ, Clemmons NS, et al. Frequency and causes of nonbattle injuries air evacuated from Operations Iraqi Freedom and Enduring Freedom, U.S. Army, 2001-2006. Am J Prev Med 2010;38(1 Suppl):S94–107.

19. Writer JV, DeFraites RF, Keep LW. Non-battle injury casualties during the Persian Gulf War and other deployments. Am J Prev Med 2000;18(3 Suppl):64–70.

20. Belmont PJ Jr, Goodman GP, Waterman B, et al. Disease and nonbattle injuries sustained by a U.S. Army Brigade Combat Team during Operation Iraqi Freedom. Mil Med 2010;175(7):469–76.

21. Goodman GP, Schoenfeld AJ, Owens BD, et al. Non-emergent orthopaedic injuries sustained by soldiers in Operation Iraqi Freedom. J Bone Joint Surg Am 2012;94(8):728–35.

22. Blank E, Owens BD, Burks R, et al. Incidence of trochanteric bursitis in the US military. Orthopedics 2012;35:e1022–7.

23. Cameron KL, Hsiao MS, Owens BD, et al. Incidence of physician-diagnosed osteoarthritis among active duty United States military service members. Arthritis Rheum 2011;63(10):2974–82.
24. Wolf JM, Dawson L, Mountcastle SB, et al. The incidence of scaphoid fracture in a military population. Injury 2009;40(12):1316–9.
25. Wolf JM, Mountcastle S, Owens BD. Incidence of carpal tunnel syndrome in the US military population. Hand (N Y) 2009;4(3):289–93.
26. Wolf JM, Sturdivant RX, Owens BD. Incidence of de Quervain's tenosynovitis in a young, active population. J Hand Surg Am 2009;34(1):112–5.
27. Scher DL, Belmont PJ Jr, Mountcastle S, et al. The incidence of primary hip osteoarthritis in active duty US military servicemembers. Arthritis Rheum 2009;61(4):468–75.
28. Scher DL, Belmont PJ Jr, Bear R, et al. The incidence of plantar fasciitis in the United States military. J Bone Joint Surg Am 2009;91(12):2867–72.
29. Scher DL, Owens BD, Sturdivant RX, et al. Incidence of joint hypermobility syndrome in a military population: impact of gender and race. Clin Orthop Relat Res 2010;468:1790–5.
30. Cameron KL, Owens BD, DeBerardino TM. Incidence of ankle sprains among active duty members of the United States Armed Services between 1998-2006. J Athl Train 2010;45(1):29–38.
31. Owens B, Mountcastle S, White D. Racial differences in tendon rupture incidence. Int J Sports Med 2007;28(7):617–20.
32. Owens BD, Dawson L, Burks R, et al. Incidence of shoulder dislocation in the United States military: demographic considerations from a high-risk population. J Bone Joint Surg Am 2009;91(4):791–6.
33. Owens BD, Mountcastle SB, Dunn WR, et al. Incidence of anterior cruciate ligament injury among active duty U.S. military servicemen and servicewomen. Mil Med 2007;172(1):90–1.
34. Wolf JM, Mountcastle S, Burks R, et al. Epidemiology of lateral and medial epicondylitis in a military population. Mil Med 2010;175(5):336–9.
35. Hsiao M, Owens BD, Burks R, et al. Incidence of acute traumatic patellar dislocation among active-duty United States military service members. Am J Sports Med 2010;38(10):1997–2004.
36. Jones JC, Burks R, Owens BD, et al. Incidence and risk factors associated with meniscal injuries among active-duty US military service members. J Athl Train 2012;47(1):67–73.
37. Knox J, Orchowski J, Scher DL, et al. The incidence of low back pain in active duty United States military service members. Spine (Phila Pa 1976) 2011;36(18):1492–500.
38. Knox JB, Orchowski JR, Owens B. Racial differences in the incidence of acute low back pain in US military service members. Spine (Phila Pa 1976) 2012;37:1688–92.
39. Ernat J, Knox J, Orchowski J, et al. Incidence and risk factors for acute low back pain in active duty infantry. Mil Med 2012;177:1348–51.
40. Hsiao MS, Cameron KL, Huh J, et al. Clavicle fractures in the United States military: Incidence and characteristics. Mil Med 2012;117(8):970–4. PMID: 22934379.
41. Arendt E, Dick R. Knee injury patterns among men and women in collegiate basketball and soccer. NCAA data and review of literature. Am J Sports Med 1995;23(6):694–701.
42. Fithian DC, Paxton EW, Stone ML, et al. Epidemiology and natural history of acute patellar dislocation. Am J Sports Med 2004;32(5):1114–21.

43. Atkin DM, Fithian DC, Marangi KS, et al. Characteristics of patients with primary acute lateral patellar dislocation and their recovery within the first 6 months of injury. Am J Sports Med 2000;28(4):472–9.

44. Sillanpaa PJ, Maenpaa HM, Mattila VM, et al. Arthroscopic surgery for primary traumatic patellar dislocation: a prospective, nonrandomized study comparing patients treated with and without acute arthroscopic stabilization with a median 7-year follow-up. Am J Sports Med 2008;36(12):2301–9.

45. Dunn WR, Lincoln AE, Hinton RY, et al. Occupational disability after hospitalization for the treatment of an injury of the anterior cruciate ligament. J Bone Joint Surg Am 2003;85-A(9):1656–66.

46. Dunn WR, Lyman S, Lincoln AE, et al. The effect of anterior cruciate ligament reconstruction on the risk of knee reinjury. Am J Sports Med 2004;32(8): 1906–14.

47. Lohmander LS, Englund PM, Dahl LL, et al. The long-term consequence of anterior cruciate ligament and meniscus injuries: osteoarthritis. Am J Sports Med 2007;35(10):1756–69.

48. Lohmander LS, Ostenberg A, Englund M, et al. High prevalence of knee osteoarthritis, pain, and functional limitations in female soccer players twelve years after anterior cruciate ligament injury. Arthritis Rheum 2004;50(10):3145–52.

49. Englund M, Lohmander LS. Risk factors for symptomatic knee osteoarthritis fifteen to twenty-two years after meniscectomy. Arthritis Rheum 2004;50(9):2811–9.

50. Kuikka PI, Pihlajamaki HK, Mattila VM. Knee injuries related to sports in young adult males during military service–incidence and risk factors. Scand J Med Sci Sports 2013;23(3):281–7.

51. Gerber JP, Williams GN, Scoville CR, et al. Persistent disability associated with ankle sprains: a prospective examination of an athletic population. Foot Ankle Int 1998;19(10):653–60.

52. Strowbridge NF, Burgess KR. Sports and training injuries in British soldiers: the Colchester Garrison Sports Injury and Rehabilitation Centre. J R Army Med Corps 2002;148(3):236–43.

53. Waterman BR, Owens BD, Davey S, et al. The epidemiology of ankle sprains in the United States. J Bone Joint Surg Am 2010;92(13):2279–84.

54. Zacchilli MA, Owens BD. Epidemiology of shoulder dislocations presenting to emergency departments in the United States. J Bone Joint Surg Am 2010; 92(3):542–9.

55. Owens BD, Duffey ML, Nelson BJ, et al. The incidence and characteristics of shoulder instability at the United States Military Academy. Am J Sports Med 2007;35(7):1168–73.

56. Waterman BR, Burns TC, McCriskin B, et al. Outcomes after Bankart repair in a military population: predictors for surgical revision and long-term disability. Arthroscopy 2014;30(2):172–7.

57. Waterman BR, et al. Trends in the diagnosis of SLAP lesions in the US military. Knee Surg Sports Traumatol Arthrosc 2013. http://dx.doi.org/10.1007/s00167-013-2798-z [Epub ahead of print]. PMID: 24318507.

58. Jerosch J, Castro WH, Assheuer J. Age-related magnetic resonance imaging morphology of the menisci in asymptomatic individuals. Arch Orthop Trauma Surg 1996;115(3-4):199–202.

59. Knapik J, Montain SJ, McGraw S, et al. Stress fracture risk factors in basic combat training. Int J Sports Med 2012;33(11):940–6.

60. Owens BD, Wolf JM, Seelig AD, et al. Risk factors for lower extremity tendinopathies in military personnel. Orthop J Sports Med 2013;1(1):1–8.

61. Brawley S, Fairbanks K, Nguyen W, et al. Sports medicine training room clinic model for the military. Mil Med 2012;177(2):135–8.
62. Masters D. Sports medicine and rehabilitation team clinic: comparative model analysis of Navy and Marine Corps Options. Falls Church (VA): Department of Defense; 2003. p. 100.
63. Rodewig C. Health of the force: action teams promote injury prevention for trainees. Army News Archives 2013 [cited 2014, January 17, 2014]. Available at: http://www.army.mil/article/94795/. Accessed 17 January, 2014.
64. Musculoskeletal action team/athletic training program solicitation number W911SF13R0026. 2013 [cited 2014]. Available at: https://www.fbo.gov/?s=opportunity&mode=form&id=0288306c4112f8826e0d46980a74f9aa&tab=core&_cview=1. Accessed 17 January, 2014.

Lower Extremity Stress Fractures in the Military

Jeremy M. Jacobs, MD[a], Kenneth L. Cameron, PhD, MPH, ATC[b], John A. Bojescul, MD[a],*

KEYWORDS

- Stress fracture • Military • Recruit • Femoral neck

KEY POINTS

- Stress fractures of the lower extremities are common among the military population and athletes.
- Modifiable risk factors include poor nutritional status, low entry-level fitness, and rapid progression of intensity and duration of exercise.
- Nonmodifiable risk factors include female sex, advanced age, and those individuals who have already sustained a stress fracture.
- Prevention is aimed at manipulating the modifiable risk factors, such as altering overall training volume and limiting distance running.
- In the soldier or athlete who presents with activity-related pain, stress fractures should be given significant consideration during the clinical evaluation.

INTRODUCTION

Stress fractures are common injuries in athletes, dancers, and military populations.[1–6] These fractures can be partial or complete fractures of bone that result from repetitive microtrauma. Bone remodeling normally occurs as a balance of osteoclastic resorption and osteoblastic production in response to physiologic stress and mechanical loads. As osteoblastic activation lags behind resorption, there is a period of time when fracture risk increases because of weakened bone.[7–9] Many individuals who sustain stress fractures can identify a sudden increase in workout intensity or duration as a precipitating factor for injury, and it is thought that gradual progressions in both exercise intensity and duration may reduce the risk of fracture.[3] As the nation has become more sedentary and overweight in recent years, the overall fitness level of military recruits has declined.[10] As a result, the rigorous physical requirements during basic combat training place the new soldier at an increased risk for sustaining several lower extremity overuse injuries; however, one of the most significant injuries

[a] Dwight David Eisenhower Army Medical Center, 300 E Hospital Road, Ft Gordon, GA 30905, USA; [b] Keller Army Community Hospital, 900 Washington Road, West Point, New York 10996, USA
* Corresponding author.
E-mail address: John.a.bojescul2.mil@mail.mil

Clin Sports Med 33 (2014) 591–613
http://dx.doi.org/10.1016/j.csm.2014.06.002
0278-5919/14/$ – see front matter Published by Elsevier Inc.

sportsmed.theclinics.com

sustained in this population is insufficiency or stress fracture.[2,3,11] The purpose of this review is to discuss the epidemiology and pathogenesis of stress fractures with a focus on reviewing the current literature on injury prevention and the assessment, diagnosis, and clinical management of low- and high-risk stress fractures within the active-duty military population.

THE BURDEN AND PATHOGENESIS OF STRESS FRACTURE INJURIES IN PHYSICALLY ACTIVE POPULATIONS
Incidence and Impact

Lower extremity stress fracture injuries disproportionately affect athletes and military service members who regularly engage in vigorous weight-bearing physical activities. Stress fractures, particularly in high-risk regions of the proximal femur, hip, and pelvis, can lead to serious injury, morbidity, and potentially long-term disability. These injuries can also negatively impact force readiness and lead to lost training time, failure to complete training requirements, and medical discharge from military service. Service members are typically at the greatest risk for stress fracture during basic combat training and initial entry-level training. Studies have reported the cumulative incidence or incidence proportion of lower extremity stress fracture during initial entry-level military training to range from 0.8% to 6.9% for men and 3.4% to 21.0% for women.[3] A recent large-scale population-based study reported stress fracture injury incidence during basic combat training to be 6.9 cases per 1000 recruits among men and 26.1 cases per 1000 recruits among women.[12]

Risk factors for lower extremity stress fracture injuries have traditionally been categorized by loci into either intrinsic (individual characteristics) or extrinsic (environmental factors external to the individual) factors. However, in order to prevent lower extremity stress fractures, it is critical to identify and focus on the modifiable risk factors associated with injury.[3] As a result, classifying risk factors by whether they are modifiable or nonmodifiable is much more relevant from a clinical and injury prevention perspective.[13] The modifiable risk factors for lower extremity stress fractures serve as important targets for injury prevention interventions. Other risk factors may be potentially modifiable. These factors can be modified under certain circumstances but might not be modifiable under others because of resource or other constraints (eg, running routes or surfaces). Nonmodifiable risk factors are equally important for identifying individuals and populations that are at the greatest risk for injury,[13] but these factors cannot be altered via intervention. In addition to establishing those that are most likely to sustain lower extremity stress fractures, nonmodifiable risk factors can also serve to inform screening guidelines and preventative measures, particularly in the presence of other modifiable risk factors. The modifiable, potentially modifiable, and nonmodifiable risk factors associated with lower extremity stress fracture are presented in **Table 1**. The remainder of this section provides an overview of the most common modifiable and nonmodifiable risk factors associated with lower extremity stress fractures.

Modifiable Risk Factors

Some of the most important modifiable risk factors for lower extremity stress fractures among individuals entering military service are poor indices of entry-level physical fitness. Many studies have demonstrated that poor entry-level aerobic fitness is associated with the subsequent risk of stress fracture, and Jones and colleagues[3] summarized several of these studies in a systematic review. Based on data from several prospective studies, individuals with the slowest entry-level run times were 2.5 to 7.7 times as likely to experience lower extremity stress fracture injuries during basic

Table 1
Modifiable, potentially modifiable, and nonmodifiable risk factors for lower extremity stress fractures

Modifiable Risk Factors	Risk Factor Loci
Entry-level Physical Fitness	
Lower aerobic fitness	Intrinsic
Lower muscle strength and endurance	Intrinsic
Poorer flexibility	Intrinsic
Biomechanical Movement Patterns	
Greater peak hip adduction angle (gait)	Intrinsic
Greater peak rear foot eversion angle (gait)	Intrinsic
Increased sagittal plane knee stiffness (gait)	Intrinsic
Increased absolute free moment (gait)	Intrinsic
Increased vertical force impact peak (gait)	Intrinsic
Increased peak positive acceleration of the tibia (gait)	Intrinsic
Increased tibial shock (gait)	Intrinsic
Increased peak vertical loading rate (gait)	Intrinsic
Increased peak vertical ground reaction force (jump landing task)	Intrinsic
Increased medial ground reaction force (jump landing task)	Intrinsic
Increased knee valgus (jump landing task)	Intrinsic
Increased knee internal rotation (jump landing task)	Intrinsic
Body Composition	
Lower body mass index	Intrinsic
Nutritional Factors	
Low serum vitamin D	Intrinsic
Low calcium	Intrinsic
Poor diet and low caloric intake relative to demands	Intrinsic
Other Health Risk Behaviors	
Smoking and tobacco use	Intrinsic
Sedentary lifestyle	Intrinsic
Amenorrhea and menstrual irregularity	Intrinsic
Footwear	
Shoe type	Extrinsic
Boot type	Extrinsic
Insoles or orthotic devices	Extrinsic
Training-Related Variables	
Rapid progression in	
Training volume	Extrinsic
Training intensity	Extrinsic
Training duration	Extrinsic
Training frequency	Extrinsic
Training distance	Extrinsic
Any combination of these variables	

(continued on next page)

Table 1 *(continued)*	
Modifiable Risk Factors	**Risk Factor Loci**
Potentially Modifiable Risk Factors	
Low bone mineral density	Intrinsic
Type of training activity/sport	Extrinsic
Training environment	
Type of running surface (eg, pavement, dirt, grass, track)	Extrinsic
Nonmodifiable Risk Factors	
Female sex	Intrinsic
Increased age	Intrinsic
White race	Intrinsic
History of lower extremity stress fractures	Intrinsic
Lower extremity morphology & anatomic factors	
High arches in the foot	Intrinsic
Genu valgum at the knee (knock-kneed)	Intrinsic
High quadriceps angle (Q angle)	Intrinsic
Leg length discrepancy	Intrinsic
Bone geometry	Intrinsic

Adapted from Jones BH, Thacker SB, Gilchrist J, et al. Prevention of lower extremity stress fractures in athletes and soldiers: a systematic review. Epidemiol Rev 2002;24:228–47.

combat training when compared with those with the fastest entry-level run times. Whether or not entry-level strength or flexibility is associated with the risk of stress fracture injuries remains unclear, as conflicting results have been reported in the literature; however, a recent prospective study suggests that knee flexor and extensor weakness may be associated with the incidence rate of lower extremity stress fractures, as this can limit the ability to dissipate force in the sagittal plane during gait and jumping tasks.[14] Studies also show that those who lead sedentary lifestyles, or do not report regularly engaging in weight-bearing physical activities before beginning basic combat training in the military, are also at increased risk for lower extremity stress fractures during initial entry-level training.[3] Furthermore, a rapid progression in total weight-bearing exercise volume, frequency, intensity, or duration within these individuals, as is typical during basic combat training, is commonly associated with lower extremity stress fractures.[15] These training-related variables are all modifiable, and appropriately managing a gradual progression and increase in exercise volume can likely mitigate the risk of lower extremity stress fractures among athletes and military personnel during the early weeks of training.

Several studies have recently focused on how biomechanical movement patterns during gait[15–21] and landing from a jump[14] might be associated with the risk for lower extremity stress fractures (see **Table 1**). These movement patterns are important because recent studies have demonstrated that movement retraining interventions might be effective in mitigating these factors and potentially the subsequent risk for lower extremity stress fractures.[22–24] Milner and colleagues[20] reported that free moment during gait, which is a measure of torque about a vertical axis at the interface of the shoe and the ground and serves as a surrogate measure of torque acting on the tibia, was associated with a history of tibial stress fracture. In a related study, Milner and colleagues[18] also reported that tibial stress fracture cases had significantly greater instantaneous and average vertical loading rates and tibial shock during gait, when compared with uninjured controls. In addition to increased loading rates and tibial shock, Milner and colleagues[19] also reported increased sagittal plane knee stiffness among tibial stress fracture cases and that increased knee stiffness was associated with increased tibial shock. The same group[16,17] subsequently reported that free moment, hip adduction angle, and rear foot eversion angle during gait were associated with a history of tibial stress fractures. Although these cross-sectional studies provide important insight into the biomechanical differences between tibial stress fracture cases and uninjured controls, because of the limitations of study design, it is not possible to determine whether these movement patterns were present before the injury or whether they were the result of the injury. Prospective studies are needed to determine the temporal relationship between preinjury biomechanical movement patterns and the subsequent risk of injury. Cameron and colleagues[14] recently reported the findings of a large prospective cohort study that examined the association between baseline preinjury biomechanical movement patterns during a jump landing task and the subsequent incidence rate of lower extremity stress fractures during 4 years of follow-up. They reported that those that went on to develop a stress fracture during follow-up had greater internal knee rotation, greater knee valgus angle, and greater peak vertical ground reaction forces. They also reported that stress fracture cases were weaker in knee flexion and extension strength, which may have contributed to increased vertical ground reaction forces in their study and the increased sagittal plane knee stiffness and tibial shock observed by Milner and colleagues[18,19] Overall, these studies suggest that patients who develop lower extremity stress fractures may exhibit specific movement patterns that place them at an increased risk for injury, and many of these movement patterns have been shown to be amenable to intervention.

Nutritional factors and body composition are also important modifiable risk factors that have been associated with lower extremity stress fracture injury. Several studies have reported that low body mass index (BMI) is an important risk factor for stress fracture injury in both men and women,[3,12,14,25] and higher BMI may be a protective factor among women during basic combat training.[12] Energy balance during intense physical activity may also be critical, particularly among women, in mitigating the risk for lower extremity stress fracture.[15,26] Adequate levels of calcium and vitamin D are essential for bone health, and inadequate intake of these nutrients has been associated with osteoporosis and osteomalacia.[15] Recent studies have also shown that inadequate levels of vitamin D and calcium may also be associated with the risk of lower extremity stress fractures.[15,27–32] Increasing BMI and vitamin D and calcium intake as well as ensuring appropriate caloric intake to achieve energy balance during periods of intense physical training may be important in mitigating the risk of lower extremity stress fracture injury.

Other modifiable health risk behaviors may also be important risk factors for lower extremity stress fracture injury. Studies have shown that tobacco use and alcohol consumption may be associated with the increased risk of lower extremity stress fracture during military training.[3,15] Also, the use of nonsteroidal antiinflammatory drugs, such as ibuprofen, may contribute to stress fracture risk and may also delay fracture healing.[15] Finally, oral contraceptive use may be a protective factor that may reduce the risk of stress fracture among women, particularly those who are amenorrheic/oligomenorrheic.[15]

Nonmodifiable Risk Factors

Several nonmodifiable risk factors for lower extremity stress fracture injuries have been identified, and these factors are important in identifying individuals and populations who are at the greatest risk of injury (see **Table 1**). Many demographic factors have been associated with the risk of lower extremity stress fractures. Studies have consistently reported that female sex is a significant risk factor for lower extremity stress fractures[3] and that women are as much as 5 times as likely to sustain a stress fracture during basic combat training when compared with men.[12] Older age has also been significantly associated with the risk of lower extremity stress fractures in numerous studies conducted in military populations.[3,12] Similarly, race other than black has been associated with an increased risk for lower extremity stress fracture injuries in several studies.[3,12] A history of lower extremity stress fractures has been associated with an increased risk of subsequent injury.[33,34] This finding highlights the importance of primary and secondary injury prevention, particularly among those with a history of prior stress fracture. Individuals with a history of stress fracture may also warrant additional screening for other modifiable risk factors before engaging in rigorous physical training. Finally, several risk factors associated with lower extremity morphology and anatomy have been examined, but most of these factors are not readily amenable to intervention.

Pathogenesis

Stress fractures have long been associated with military training programs. Many investigators have postulated the cause of stress fractures. Johnson[35] reported on a large biopsy series in which it was postulated that an accelerated remodeling phase was likely responsible for the formation of stress fractures. However, Freidenberg[36] proposed that stress fractures may be a nonunited fracture caused by the absence of significant callous at the fracture site. Stanitski and colleagues[37] described abundant new subperiosteal bone formation in 2 biopsy specimens. They also note that "subthreshold mechanical insults summate beyond the stress bearing capacity of the bone"[37] and that the onset of fracture is a combination of the stress duration and ability of bone to repair itself (**Box 1**).

ASSESSMENT AND DIAGNOSIS OF STRESS FRACTURE INJURIES
Clinical Evaluation

Patients will report the insidious onset of pain over a period of weeks, which typically corresponds to a particular increase in activity level or endurance training. This pain may be relieved by periods of rest and immobilization. It is important to complete a thorough medical history including diet and endocrine disorders, with an important focus on menstrual history in the female athlete. Physical examination is significant for localized tenderness to palpation when suspected injury is within a superficial bone, such as the anterior tibia. Likewise, erythema and edema may be evidence of underlying pathology. For deep structures where a stress fracture is suspected, gentle range-of-motion

---

Box 1
Pathogenesis of stress fracture

1. Increased external and muscular forces

2. Resorption and remodeling

3. Focal microfractures

4. Endosteal and periosteal reaction, stress fracture

5. Linear fracture that can advance to displaced fracture

exercises will elicit pain. Alignment and biomechanical evaluation must be examined to identify factors placing patients at an increased risk for fatigue fractures.[38]

Imaging

Plain radiographs are the initial imaging modality of choice, as they are readily available and inexpensive. Subtle signs may preclude the need for advanced imaging, such as blurring of the cortex and periosteal reaction, which may be evident. More mature stress fractures may present with a cortical lucency, frank fracture line, or evidence of new callus formation.[39] It is important to note that radiographic signs may lag weeks behind clinical complaints. In the case of occult fracture, 3-phase bone scan with technetium 99 is very helpful, as this study has high sensitivity early in the process of stress fracture. The third phase will typically illustrate increased intensity, which sets apart boney injury from localized soft tissue injuries, such as contusion or muscle strain.[40] Scintigraphy is not particularly specific and has been noted to have a false-positive rate nearing 50%. Magnetic resonance imaging (MRI) has been noted to be as sensitive as a bone scan but more specific.[41] Fluid-sensitive sequences can show periosteal and marrow edema as well as localized soft tissue inflammation within 24 hours, whereas a bone scan may show increased uptake in as early as 48 hours. Cortical irregularities can be detected, and fractures will present as a characteristic linear hypointense signal.

TREATMENT OF COMMON HIGH-RISK STRESS FRACTURES
Femoral Neck

Although stress fractures of the femoral neck make up only 10% of all stress fractures, the results can lead to long-term disability as a result of pain, nonunion, and osteonecrosis of the femoral head.[42,43] This injury is particularly devastating for the new military recruit who may be discharged from military service with a prolonged recovery. Talbot's case series of 20 military recruits in the United Kingdom demonstrated a 40% medical discharge rate, and Johansson found that 60% of athletes sustaining displaced femoral neck stress fractures (FNSF) failed to return to preinjury activity levels.[44,45] Patients typically present with anterior groin pain and an inability to bear weight. Tenderness to palpation is not common, but pain at the extremes of internal and external rotation will elicit discomfort.

Radiographic examination includes routine pelvis and hip views. Early in the process, radiographs are unimpressive; MRI may be warranted if symptoms fail to improve. Carey and colleagues[46] demonstrated that military recruits who sustain FNSF have a high prevalence of radiographic findings suggestive of femoroacetabular impingement. MRI will demonstrate bony edema (most commonly to the compression side of the femoral neck), and a fracture line may be present. **Fig. 1** demonstrates typical findings when investigating FNSF.

If patients present early, nonoperative treatment is often successful. If a FNSF is suspected, immediate non–weight bearing (NWB) is implemented while appropriate imaging studies can be completed. A minimum of 4 to 6 weeks of NWB is continued; as symptoms resolve, progressive weight bearing can be slowly accelerated based on symptoms and clinical examination in those patients with evidence of stress reaction on MRI. Typically patients are back to light-impact activities at 3 to 4 months. There is concern for tension-sided femoral neck fractures, as these have a higher propensity to propagate to displaced fractures. It is recommended that all tension-sided fractures as well as compression-sided fractures that comprise greater than 50% of the neck width should undergo percutaneous cannulated screw placement to prevent

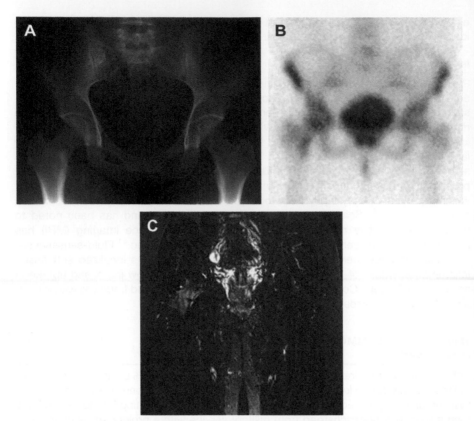

Fig. 1. Imaging of a 26-year-old female recruit with a 4-week history of atraumatic right hip pain worsened with activity during basic training. She was made non–weight bearing for 6 weeks and completed a graded progression back to baseline activity without long-term sequelae.

displacement.[47] Patients should remain NWB for 6 weeks and then progress to full weight bearing over the next 6 weeks.[38] Displaced FNSF should be urgently managed with open reduction and internal fixation (ORIF) and typically takes longer for union. Evans and colleagues[48] reviewed 6 cases of displaced fractures in Royal Marine recruits and noted a 100% union rate at an average of 11 months. Fifty percent of the cases took greater than 12 months for radiographic evidence of union.[48]

Femoral Shaft

Fatigue fractures of the femoral shaft are less common than femoral neck fractures but more common in military recruits and endurance athletes. Orava[49] noted a 3% incidence of femoral shaft stress fractures, and others have quoted rates nearing 20% of all stress fractures.[50] Niva and colleagues[51] noted an 18% incidence rate of proximal shaft fractures among 185 fatigue injuries in Finnish military recruits. Fractures of the proximal third shaft are most common. Patients will present with vague thigh pain but may also note referred hip or knee pain. There is rarely loss of hip range of motion, unlike femoral neck lesions, but similar complaints with weight bearing. The fulcrum test as described by Johnson and colleagues[50] is highly correlated with stress injuries and is executed by placing the examiner's arm beneath the midshaft of the thigh and providing a dorsally (posteriorly) directed force about the distal femur. A positive test is indicated by exacerbation and recreation of pain. As seen in **Fig. 2**, plain films are often without irregularities; but advanced imaging will demonstrate evidence of stress fracture.

Conservative treatment of femoral shaft fractures is often successful, and nonoperative treatment mirrors that for femoral neck fractures. A period of NWB is necessary and followed by progressive rehabilitation after successful evidence of radiographic healing. Weishaar and colleagues[52] discussed the conservative management of 2 US Military Academy cadets who sustained femoral shaft stress fractures and both returned to full athletic activities at 12 weeks without complication. Displaced fractures of the femoral shaft are rare and should be treated urgently. Salminen and colleagues[53] discussed 10 displaced femoral shaft stress fractures over a 20-year period at a national military hospital and noted an incidence of 1.5 per 100,000 person-years of military service. The investigators noted 90% had antecedent thigh or knee pain, and only one displaced fracture occurred in the proximal third shaft. These fractures were treated based on the location and fracture characteristics just as an acute fracture. Five patients underwent intramedullary nailing, 4 with dynamic compression plating and one with a condylar blade plate; the average time to union was 3.5 months.[53]

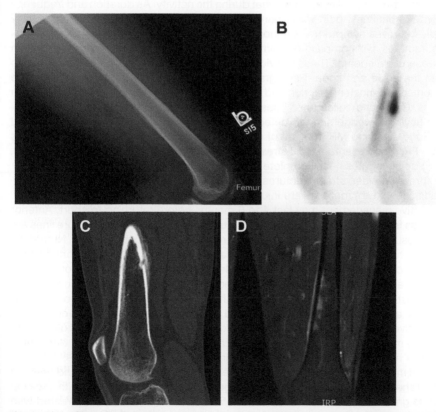

Fig. 2. Plain films demonstrate a subtle posterior periosteal reaction. Bone scan and MRI localize the lesion, and a selected computed tomography cut illustrates incomplete posterior cortical stress fracture in an 18-year-old man with left thigh pain at the completion of basic training.

Tibia

Tibial stress fractures account for most of the lower extremity fractures and make up 50% of all reported stress fractures.[54–56] These fractures are common in both the athletic and military communities. A prospective study of US Marine Corps recruits found that tibial stress fractures made up 73% percent of the initial fatigue fracture diagnoses, and Giladi and colleagues[57] noted an abnormally high incidence of 71% in Israeli Defense Force infantry recruits.[58] Most tibial stress fractures occur along the posteromedial cortex in a transverse direction and result from repetitive compressive forces, notable in distance running. On the other hand, anterior tibial stress fractures pose a significant threat to the patient and are more common in repetitive jumping and leaping activities. These fractures are thought to be a result of tensile forces placed on the anterior cortex by the strong posterior musculature and have a high propensity for prolonged healing, nonunion, and completion of fracture.[59] Investigators have demonstrated an incidence of 4.6% for anterior tibial stress fractures.[60] Kilcoyne and colleagues[61] demonstrated positive outcomes for US Naval Academy midshipmen 10 years after injury. There were no significant limitations in completing military training, and no patients were separated from the military as a result of sustaining a tibial stress fracture based on long-term follow-up.[61]

On clinical presentation, most patients will complain of activity-related pain that is worse at start-up and relieves somewhat during the activity. As duration and frequency of exercise continues, pain will continue to increase. Cessation of offending activity typically improves symptoms. A minority of patients, who present with anterior tibial stress fractures, will complain of point tenderness at the site of injury and may even have observable edema. These individuals will normally maintain full range of motion of both the ankle and knee. Radiographs are normal initially but may demonstrate posteromedial periosteal reaction and callus formation in late presenting compression fractures. Rettig and colleagues[62] described tension-sided stress fractures as radiographs having a wedge shaped defect in the middle third of the anterolateral tibial shaft. Bone scan and MRI may be of use if the diagnosis and clinical presentation is unclear. **Fig. 3** represents a tibial stress fracture that appears benign on radiographs, but MRI demonstrates near-complete fracture of the proximal tibial diaphysis.

Compression-sided stress fractures generally respond to a period of rest and activity modification, with more severe injuries requiring a short course of immobilization. Conservative management may last 4 to 6 months before returning to sport. Anterior tibial stress fractures and posterior tibial fractures that have widening fracture lines are likely to result in delayed or nonunion and require surgical intervention. Numerous treatments have been proposed. Nonsurgical treatments of delayed unions include external electromagnetic stimulation and pulsed ultrasound. Rettig and colleagues[62] demonstrated healing in 7 of 8 patients treated with pulsed electromagnetic field therapy and rest for an average of 8.7 months after initiation of treatment, and most patients were able to return to competition at 1 year. Rue and colleagues[63] completed a prospective, randomized, double-blind clinical study investigating pulsed ultrasound in US Navy midshipmen and found no significant reduction in healing time. Continuing research is needed to elucidate the effectiveness of noninvasive therapies.

Surgical management is indicated for acutely displaced tibial fractures and pending or established nonunions. Green and colleagues[59] treated 5 nonunions with excision and bone grafting, and all had union within 5 months. One patient was treated with excision alone and failed to unite during the follow-up period. Critics of this method note donor site morbidity when using iliac crest and the requirement of postoperative immobilization until evidence of union. Borens and colleagues[64] presented promising

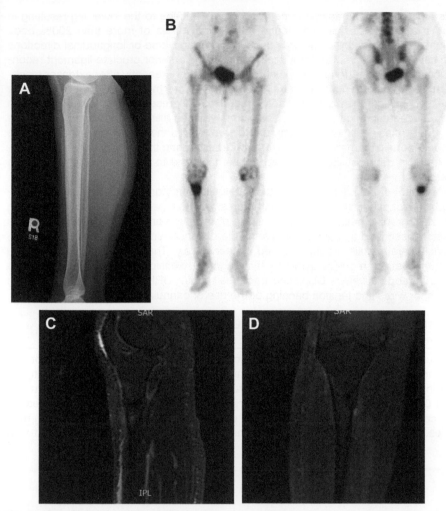

Fig. 3. Plain films of a tibial stress fracture demonstrate normal cortical margins without evidence of fracture or periosteal reaction. Bone scan shows increased uptake to the proximal tibia, and MRI clearly defines a near-complete fracture of the tibial metadiaphysis. The patient was treated conservatively with immobilization and NWB as symptoms slowly resolved over 12 weeks.

results with anterior tension band plating in 4 cases found in high-performance female athletes. Each fracture was grafted with demineralized bone matrix; all fractures united, with return to full activity at a mean of 10 weeks. Chang and Harris[65] presented 5 cases of US Army servicemen who underwent reamed intramedullary nailing for chronic anterior tibial stress fractures and noted good to excellent results in all. At this time, intramedullary fixation is the preferred treatment method for chronic anterior tibial stress fractures.[38]

Patella

Although a very rare fatigue injury, stress fractures of the patella require special attention because of the significant disability of extensor mechanism disruption. The patella acts as a fulcrum to transmit force from the quadriceps to the lower leg resulting in knee extension and has been found to transmit forces of more than 200% body weight.[66] Patellar fatigue fractures can occur in transverse or longitudinal directions and have been found after total knee arthroplasty, anterior cruciate ligament reconstruction using bone-tendon-bone autograft, and more recently after extensor mechanism repair with transosseous tunnels.[67–70] They are most common in endurance athletes. Patients with patellar stress fractures will present with anterior knee pain and reduced tolerance to deep knee flexion, whereas displaced transverse fractures may present as an extensor mechanism disruption. To the authors' knowledge, there are no reports of primary patellar stress fractures among the military population; however, **Fig. 4** demonstrates increased uptake localized to the patella consistent with stress fracture.

Treatment of fatigue fractures of the patella depends on the fracture pattern. Nondisplaced longitudinal or transverse fractures require a period of knee immobilization until radiographic healing is evident. Close observation and follow-up is required, as Devas[71] described an early case of a middle-distance runner who sustained a longitudinal lateral patellar fracture treated conservatively. Three months after presentation, the patient required symptomatic fragment excision, and fibrous union was found intraoperatively.[71] Displaced fractures require ORIF in standard fashion with Kirschner wires and tension banding or the use of cannulated compression screws.

TREATMENT OF COMMON LOW-RISK STRESS FRACTURES
Calcaneus

Fractures of the calcaneus may be the most common stress fracture of the foot and are most common among distance runners, the elderly as insufficiency fractures, and in military recruits. Among new recruits, rates of calcaneal involvement range from 0.5% to 43.0% of all stress fractures sustained during training.[72–74] Greaney and colleagues[58] found it to be the most common stress fracture of the foot in their series. Clinical presentation typically consists of heel or ankle pain worsened with

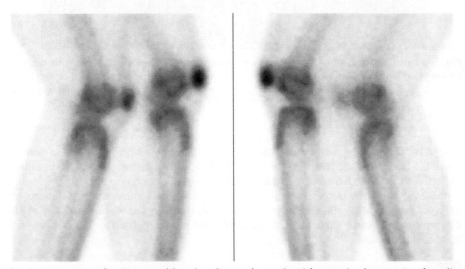

Fig. 4. Bone scan of a 25-year-old male advanced recruit with anterior knee pain after distance runs who was treated with a course of immobilization and subsequent resolution of symptoms.

activity and may have failed prior conservative treatment by primary care. Radiographs commonly show a characteristic sclerotic line superiorly in the posterior third of the calcaneus after a few weeks from the onset of symptoms (**Fig. 5**A). Recently, Sormaala and colleagues[75] presented findings on 30 calcaneal stress fractures in Finnish military recruits and found 56% occurred in the posterior, 18% in the middle, and 26% in the anterior portions of the calcaneus. It is important to suspect calcaneal stress fractures on clinical examination. Bone scan and MRI may be quite useful, as only 15% of radiographs showed evidence of fracture (see **Fig. 5**B, C).[75] Treatment consists of discontinuation of the offending activity with a course of NWB immobilization. Most patients will return to activities after months of light duty, and some military careers may be cut short. Although calcaneus fractures are common, complete and displaced calcaneal stress fractures are rare.

Tarsal Navicular

Stress fractures of the tarsal navicular bone are uncommon injuries, and most are seen in elite athletes and dancers participating in sports requiring sprinting and abrupt changes in direction. Reported rates in the military have historically ranged from 1% to 3%.[57,58,76–78] Patients will present with activity-related pain to the dorsal aspect of the midfoot, and delayed diagnosis is not uncommon. Maneuvers such as resisted plantar-flexion and jumping on the affected limb will often exacerbate pain.

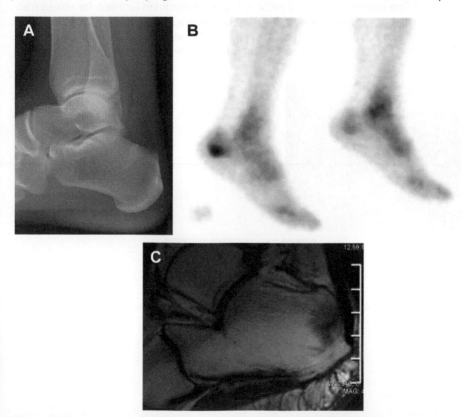

Fig. 5. Radiograph demonstrates a common pattern of calcaneal stress fracture with increased opacity to the posterosuperior margin of the calcaneus. Bone scan and MRI show a different stress fracture located at the inferior aspect of the calcaneal tuberosity.

Radiographs may be inconclusive initially and necessitate the use of advanced imaging. Stress fractures of the tarsal navicular commonly occur in the central one-third and are oriented in the sagittal plain (**Fig. 6**).

Treatment of navicular stress fractures remains in favor of nonoperative treatment with a 6-week period of NWB and immobilization. Khan and colleagues[79] reported on 86 clinical stress fractures, and 86% of patients treated with NWB cast immobilization returned to sport compared with 26% who continued weight bearing and limited activity. Fifteen patients in the latter group required at least one operation. Some investigators propose that ORIF with or without bone grafting may return the athlete faster, but Saxena and Fullem[80] demonstrated no significant difference between surgical and conservative measures. ORIF with bone grafting has shown favorable results in both primary and delayed union groups.[79–82] A 2010 meta-analysis by Torg and colleagues[83] found that there was no significant difference in outcomes for NWB cast immobilization and surgery. Thus, the investigators concluded that conservative treatment should remain the standard of care.

Metatarsals

Fractures of the metatarsals have long been associated with military service and marching when Briethaupt[84] described Prussian soldiers with swollen and painful feet after completing long marches. It has subsequently been described as "march foot."[84,85] The second metatarsal neck is the most common location for stress fractures; the third and fourth metatarsals may be involved; the proximal fifth metatarsal stress fracture is less common. **Fig. 7** demonstrates early and late radiographic findings of a third metatarsal fracture. Stress injury to the first metatarsal is uncommon

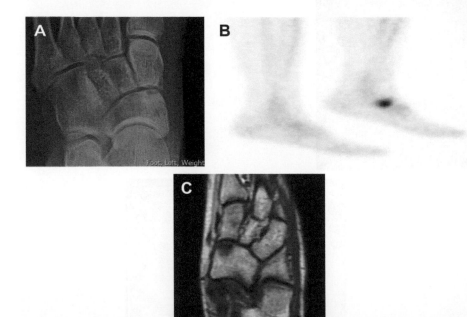

Fig. 6. A 20-year-old female recruit who presented with a 6-week history of mild midfoot pain noted only during endurance runs. Sclerosis to the medial distal aspect is noted on plain films, and bone scan and MRI confirm diagnosis of stress fracture.

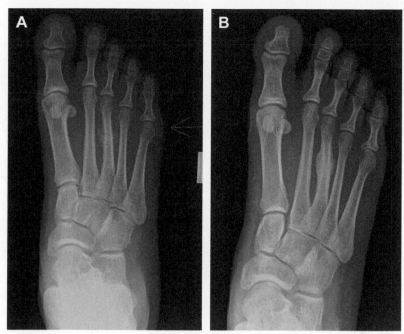

Fig. 7. Images of a 21-year-old national guardsman who complained of activity-related foot pain and dorsal edema throughout 12 weeks of basic training. (*A*) Early callous formation. (*B*) A clinically healed third metatarsal stress fracture. The patient returned to full activity 2 months after the completion of basic training.

and thought to be protected by its relative mobility.[86] The relative immobility of the second metatarsal may place this ray prone to injury. Donahue and Sharkey[87] have shown that the mean peak strain in the second metatarsal is twice that experienced by the fifth metatarsal and simulated muscle fatigue significantly increases this strain as does plantar fasciotomy.[87] Soldiers and athletes will typically complain of forefoot pain and may likely be able to localize the pain to a given metatarsal. Referral to an orthopedic provider typically occurs after a trial of conservative management by the primary care team. Treatment of the second to fourth metatarsal (MT) injuries consists of 4 weeks of immobilization in a short-leg NWB cast, a walking cast, or walking boot tailored to each patient's needs.

Special consideration is paid to the fifth metatarsal stress fractures. These injuries are common within jumping sports and have a tendency for delayed union or nonunion requiring operative intervention.[88] Patients will complain of lateral foot pain worse with running and jumping, and prodromal symptoms should provide a clue to the diagnosis. Radiographs may show a cortical lucency to the plantar aspect of the fifth metatarsal just distal to the tuberosity and incomplete callus. In cases of delayed presentation or completion of stress fracture, the medullary canal may be obliterated by sclerotic bone. **Fig. 8** demonstrates the progression from prodromal complaint to acute fracture and finally to healed stress fracture. Treatment depends on the stage at presentation, and those with short duration and no radiographic evidence of fracture can be treated conservatively with metatarsal bracing and limited weight bearing. Six weeks of cast immobilization or operative fixation is an acceptable treatment of patients with prolonged pain or radiographic evidence of fracture. Intra-medullary fixation is normally achieved with screw fixation, which is countersunk to

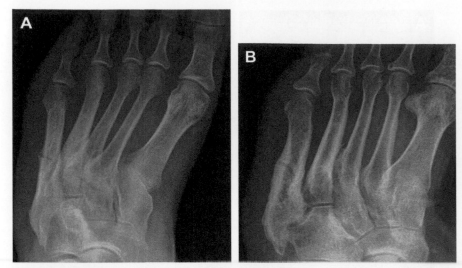

Fig. 8. Radiographs of an early, late, and healed fifth metatarsal shaft fracture in a 28-year-old active-duty soldier.

reduce soft tissue irritation. Delayed unions and those showing intramedullary sclerosis may require curettage. DeLee and colleagues[89] reported excellent results in 10 athletes in which intramedullary fixation was used to treat diaphyseal stress fractures and found that all fractures united, and the athletes returned to sport on an average of 8.5 weeks.[89]

Miscellaneous Stress Fractures

Other recognized sites of stress fractures in the lower extremity include the medial malleolus, talus, and great toe sesamoids. Upper extremity stress fractures are very rare and can occur in individuals completing repetitive lifting tasks, such as weightlifting and rifle drill training.[90,91] Honor guards are popular in the military, and some groups may practice for multiple hours per day reaching rates of 100 rotations per minute using the rifle. Stress fractures of the ulna have been noted in this unique population at a higher incidence than the general population.[92] Stress fractures of the medial malleolus and talus can occur with repetitive ankle dorsiflexion caused by impingement and are rare injuries. Fractures typically occur at the intersection of the tibial plafond and malleolus, exiting vertically or obliquely.[93] The lateral process of the talus is also prone to injury with forceful supination of the foot.[38] Imaging including plain films, bone scan, and MRI may be used. These fractures tend to respond to NWB cast immobilization, whereas return to activity can be accelerated with ORIF[94] of medial malleolar fractures. Both operative and conservative management have good outcomes and return-to-sport rates. Sesamoid fractures of the great toe occur from repetitive dorsiflexion exercises of the first ray (**Fig. 9**). These injuries respond to NWB cast immobilization. Symptomatic fibrous unions can occur and may be treated with excision.[95]

THE PREVENTION OF LOWER EXTREMITY STRESS FRACTURES

Although several promising modifiable and potentially modifiable risk factors for lower extremity stress fracture injuries have been identified and several interventions targeting these risk factors have been proposed, few have been adequately evaluated in the

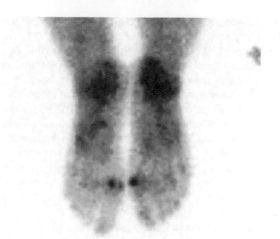

Fig. 9. Increased uptake within the bilateral hallux sesamoids in a 29-year-old active-duty soldier with normal plain radiographs. Patient was given light-duty limitations and did not run for 6 weeks with resolutions of activity-related great toe pain.

scientific literature.[3,15] The purpose of this section is to provide an overview of the existing evidence supporting primary and secondary injury prevention interventions for lower extremity stress fracture injuries.

Primary Injury Prevention

In a systematic review, Jones and colleagues[3] summarized 9 studies that evaluated the efficacy of primary injury prevention interventions in reducing the incidence of lower extremity stress fracture injuries in military populations. The studies examined interventions that consisted of modifications to the physical training program or the footwear used by Army and Marine Corps recruits during basic combat training. Few of the studies examined reported statistically or clinically significant reductions in lower extremity stress fractures and those that did typically had low overall-quality scores. More recently, studies have demonstrated that limiting running distance and overall training volume may significantly reduce but not eliminate the risk of lower extremity stress fractures in military training populations,[15] particularly as more sedentary and less physically fit individuals enter military service.

As noted previously, lower extremity biomechanical movement patterns that place individuals at an increased risk for lower extremity stress fractures may be important targets for injury prevention interventions. Recent studies have demonstrated that movement retraining interventions might be effective in mitigating these factors and potentially the subsequent risk for lower extremity stress fractures.[22–24] Crowell and Davis[23] reported that a 2-week (8 sessions) gait retraining intervention resulted in significant reductions in peak positive acceleration of the tibia, vertical force impact peak, and average and instantaneous vertical force loading rates immediately following the intervention and at the time of a 1-month postintervention assessment. Decreases in tibial acceleration (50%) and reductions in vertical force loading rate (30%) and vertical force impact peak (20%) seemed to be clinically significant; however, whether these changes are permanent or whether they actually result in reduced incidence rates of lower extremity stress fractures remain unclear. Regardless, these data suggest that movement retraining interventions that target high-risk biomechanical movement patterns may play an important role in the primary prevention of lower extremity stress fractures.

Dietary interventions focused on maintaining energy balance during rigorous physical activity and ensuring that adequate calcium and vitamin D are consumed may also be important primary prevention interventions for lower extremity stress fractures. A recent large randomized controlled trail examining the effectiveness of calcium and vitamin D supplementation in reducing the risk of stress fractures in female Navy recruits reported a statistically significant 20% reduction in those that received the intervention compared with the control (placebo) group.[27] The investigators noted that this relatively low-cost, low-risk intervention could significantly reduce morbidity and financial costs associated with lower extremity stress fractures in female recruits. Whether or not vitamin D supplementation in the absence of calcium supplementation or supplementation in men is an effective intervention to reduce the incidence of stress fractures remains unclear. A recent review and meta-analysis suggest that vitamin D supplementation may only be effective in preventing stress fractures when it is administered in combination with calcium supplements.[96,97]

Improving preaccession physical fitness levels and engaging in moderate-intensity weight-bearing physical activities that include jumping and resistance exercises several times a week can increase bone mineral density and may offer a preventive effect, particularly in high-risk recruits. Research suggests that mechanical loading, in appropriate volume and intensity, can improve bone qualities and injury resilience[98]; however, studies have yet to systematically evaluate the effectiveness of a carefully developed and monitored exercise program in reducing the risk of lower extremity stress fracture injuries in military recruits.[15] As a result, this should be an important target for future injury prevention research.

Secondary Injury Prevention

Because individuals with a history of lower extremity stress fractures are much more likely to sustain a subsequent stress fracture in the future, these individuals should be identified for additional injury screening before accession. A careful evaluation of the modifiable and other nonmodifiable risk factors associated with lower extremity stress fractures is warranted in these individuals. In particular, additional screening should focus on women with a low BMI and those that may have a history of menstrual irregularity. Screening for serum vitamin D concentrations (eg, 25-(OH)-D) might also be warranted in individuals with a history of a prior stress fracture before engaging in a rigorous physical activity program. Individuals with low serum vitamin D concentrations might benefit from dietary interventions or supplementation, and women with menstrual irregularities might benefit from low-dose oral contraceptives to reduce their risk for lower extremity stress fractures during initial entry-level military training.[15] Individuals with a history of lower extremity stress fractures might also benefit from additional biomechanical movement screening to identify high-risk movement patterns that may be addressed through movement training interventions as noted earlier. Regardless, individuals with a history of lower extremity stress fractures should garner additional scrutiny before engaging in a rigorous weight-bearing physical training program.

SUMMARY

Stress fractures of the lower extremities are common among the military population and, more specifically, military recruits who partake in basic training. Both intrinsic and extrinsic factors play a role in the development of these injuries, and it is important to identify those individuals at risk early in their military careers. Some of these factors are modifiable, so they may become preventable injuries. It is important to reiterate that one stress fracture places the soldier at risk for future stress fractures; but the first injury should not be reason enough for separation from the military, as literature would support no long-term deficits from properly treated stress fractures. Early in the process, radiographic analysis is typically normal; continued pain may warrant advanced imaging, such as scintigraphy or MRI. Most stress fractures that are caught early are amendable to nonoperative management consisting of a period of immobilization and NWB followed by progressive rehabilitation to preinjury levels. Complete or displaced fractures may require operative intervention as do tension-sided FNSF. Improving dietary and preaccession physical fitness levels may play a role in reducing the incidence of stress fractures in the active-duty military population. It is important to keep in mind when evaluating soldiers and athletes who present with activity-related pain that stress fractures are not uncommon and should be given significant consideration.

REFERENCES

1. Almeida SA, Williams KM, Shaffer RA, et al. Epidemiological patterns of musculoskeletal injuries and physical training. Med Sci Sports Exerc 1999;31(8): 1176–82.
2. Jones BH, Cowan DN, Tomlinson JP, et al. Epidemiology of injuries associated with physical training among young men in the army. Med Sci Sports Exerc 1993;25(2):197–203.
3. Jones BH, Thacker SB, Gilchrist J, et al. Prevention of lower extremity stress fractures in athletes and soldiers: a systematic review. Epidemiol Rev 2002; 24(2):228–47.
4. Kelly EW, Jonson SR, Cohen ME, et al. Stress fractures of the pelvis in female navy recruits: an analysis of possible mechanisms of injury. Mil Med 2000; 165(2):142–6.
5. Rauh MJ, Macera CA, Trone DW, et al. Epidemiology of stress fracture and lower-extremity overuse injury in female recruits. Med Sci Sports Exerc 2006; 38(9):1571–7.
6. Shaffer RA, Rauh MJ, Brodine SK, et al. Predictors of stress fracture susceptibility in young female recruits. Am J Sports Med 2006;34(1):108–15.
7. Li GP, Zhang SD, Chen G, et al. Radiographic and histologic analyses of stress fracture in rabbit tibias. Am J Sports Med 1985;13(5):285–94.
8. McBryde AM Jr. Stress fractures in runners. Clin Sports Med 1985;4(4):737–52.
9. Roub LW, Gumerman LW, Hanley EN Jr, et al. Bone stress: a radionuclide imaging perspective. Radiology 1979;132(2):431–8.
10. Hsu LL, Nevin RL, Tobler SK, et al. Trends in overweight and obesity among 18-year-old applicants to the United States military, 1993-2006. J Adolesc Health 2007;41(6):610–2.
11. Jones BH, Bovee MW, Harris JM, et al. Intrinsic risk factors for exercise-related injuries among male and female army trainees. Am J Sports Med 1993;21(5): 705–10.
12. Knapik J, Montain SJ, McGraw S, et al. Stress fracture risk factors in basic combat training. Int J Sports Med 2012;33(11):940–6.
13. Cameron KL. Commentary: time for a paradigm shift in conceptualizing risk factors in sports injury research. J Athl Train 2010;45(1):58–60.
14. Cameron KL, Peck KY, Owens BD, et al. Biomechanical risk factors for lower extremity stress fracture. Orthop J Sports Med 2013;1(4 Suppl 1).
15. Friedl KE, Evans RK, Moran DS. Stress fracture and military medical readiness: bridging basic and applied research. Med Sci Sports Exerc 2008;40(11 Suppl): S609–22.

16. Milner CE, Hamill J, Davis IS. Distinct hip and rearfoot kinematics in female runners with a history of tibial stress fracture. J Orthop Sports Phys Ther 2010;40(2): 59–66.
17. Pohl MB, Mullineaux DR, Milner CE, et al. Biomechanical predictors of retrospective tibial stress fractures in runners. J Biomech 2008;41(6):1160–5.
18. Milner CE, Ferber R, Pollard CD, et al. Biomechanical factors associated with tibial stress fracture in female runners. Med Sci Sports Exerc 2006;38(2):323–8.
19. Milner CE, Hamill J, Davis I. Are knee mechanics during early stance related to tibial stress fracture in runners? Clin Biomech (Bristol, Avon) 2007;22(6):697–703.
20. Milner CE, Davis IS, Hamill J. Free moment as a predictor of tibial stress fracture in distance runners. J Biomech 2006;39(15):2819–25.
21. Bennell K, Crossley K, Jayarajan J, et al. Ground reaction forces and bone parameters in females with tibial stress fracture. Med Sci Sports Exerc 2004;36(3): 397–404.
22. Crowell HP, Milner CE, Hamill J, et al. Reducing impact loading during running with the use of real-time visual feedback. J Orthop Sports Phys Ther 2010;40(4): 206–13.
23. Crowell HP, Davis IS. Gait retraining to reduce lower extremity loading in runners. Clin Biomech (Bristol, Avon) 2011;26(1):78–83.
24. Davis IS. Gait retraining in runners. Orthopaedic Practice 2005;17(2):8–13.
25. Beck TJ, Ruff CB, Mourtada FA, et al. Dual-energy X-ray absorptiometry derived structural geometry for stress fracture prediction in male U.S. Marine Corps recruits. J Bone Miner Res 1996;11(5):645–53.
26. Loucks AB, Thuma JR. Luteinizing hormone pulsatility is disrupted at a threshold of energy availability in regularly menstruating women. J Clin Endocrinol Metab 2003;88(1):297–311.
27. Lappe J, Cullen D, Haynatzki G, et al. Calcium and vitamin d supplementation decreases incidence of stress fractures in female navy recruits. J Bone Miner Res 2008;23(5):741–9.
28. Lutz LJ, Karl JP, Rood JC, et al. Vitamin D status, dietary intake, and bone turnover in female soldiers during military training: a longitudinal study. J Int Soc Sports Nutr 2012;9(1):38.
29. Moran DS, Heled Y, Arbel Y, et al. Dietary intake and stress fractures among elite male combat recruits. J Int Soc Sports Nutr 2012;9(1):6.
30. Sonneville KR, Gordon CM, Kocher MS, et al. Vitamin D, calcium, and dairy intakes and stress fractures among female adolescents. Arch Pediatr Adolesc Med 2012;166(7):595–600.
31. Givon U, Friedman E, Reiner A, et al. Stress fractures in the Israeli defense forces from 1995 to 1996. Clin Orthop Relat Res 2000;(373):227–32.
32. Ruohola JP, Laaksi I, Ylikomi T, et al. Association between serum 25(OH)D concentrations and bone stress fractures in Finnish young men. J Bone Miner Res 2006;21(9):1483–8.
33. Milgrom C, Giladi M, Chisin R, et al. The long-term follow-up of soldiers with stress fractures. Am J Sports Med 1985;13(6):398–400.
34. Giladi M, Milgrom C, Kashtan H, et al. Recurrent stress fractures in military recruits. One-year follow-up of 66 recruits. J Bone Joint Surg Br 1986;68(3): 439–41.
35. Johnson LC. Histogenesis of stress fractures. Armed Forces Institute of Pathology Annual Lectures. 1963.
36. Stanitski CL, McMaster JH, Scranton PE. On the nature of stress fractures. Am J Sports Med 1978;6(6):391–6.

37. Friedenberg ZB. Fatigue fractures of the tibia. Clin Orthop Relat Res 1971;76: 111–5.
38. Boden BP, Osbahr DC. High-risk stress fractures: evaluation and treatment. J Am Acad Orthop Surg 2000;8(6):344–53.
39. Daffner RH, Pavlov H. Stress fractures: current concepts. AJR Am J Roentgenol 1992;159(2):245–52.
40. Prather JL, Nusynowitz ML, Snowdy HA, et al. Scintigraphic findings in stress fractures. J Bone Joint Surg Am 1977;59(7):869–74.
41. Gaeta M, Minutoli F, Scribano E, et al. CT and MR imaging findings in athletes with early tibial stress injuries: comparison with bone scintigraphy findings and emphasis on cortical abnormalities. Radiology 2005;235(2):553–61.
42. Fullerton LR Jr. Femoral neck stress fractures. Sports Med 1990;9(3):192–7.
43. Shin AY, Gillingham BL. Fatigue fractures of the femoral neck in athletes. J Am Acad Orthop Surg 1997;5(6):293–302.
44. Johansson C, Ekenman I, Tornkvist H, et al. Stress fractures of the femoral neck in athletes. The consequence of a delay in diagnosis. Am J Sports Med 1990; 18(5):524–8.
45. Talbot JC, Cox G, Townend M, et al. Femoral neck stress fractures in military personnel–a case series. J R Army Med Corps 2008;154(1):47–50.
46. Carey T, Key C, Oliver D, et al. Prevalence of radiographic findings consistent with femoroacetabular impingement in military personnel with femoral neck stress fractures. J Surg Orthop Adv 2013;22(1):54–8.
47. Aro H, Dahlstrom S. Conservative management of distraction-type stress fractures of the femoral neck. J Bone Joint Surg Br 1986;68(1):65–7.
48. Evans JT, Guyver PM, Kassam AM, et al. Displaced femoral neck stress fractures in Royal Marine recruits–management and results of operative treatment. J R Nav Med Serv 2012;98(2):3–5.
49. Orava S. Stress fractures. Br J Sports Med 1980;14(1):40–4.
50. Johnson AW, Weiss CB Jr, Wheeler DL. Stress fractures of the femoral shaft in athletes–more common than expected. A new clinical test. Am J Sports Med 1994;22(2):248–56.
51. Niva MH, Kiuru MJ, Haataja R, et al. Fatigue injuries of the femur. J Bone Joint Surg Br 2005;87(10):1385–90.
52. Weishaar MD, McMillian DM, Moore JH. Identification and management of 2 femoral shaft stress injuries. J Orthop Sports Phys Ther 2005;35(10): 665–73.
53. Salminen ST, Pihlajamaki HK, Visuri TI, et al. Displaced fatigue fractures of the femoral shaft. Clin Orthop Relat Res 2003;(409):250–9.
54. Matheson GO, Clement DB, McKenzie DC, et al. Stress fractures in athletes. A study of 320 cases. Am J Sports Med 1987;15(1):46–58.
55. Verma RB, Sherman O. Athletic stress fractures: part I. History, epidemiology, physiology, risk factors, radiography, diagnosis, and treatment. Am J Orthop (Belle Mead NJ) 2001;30(11):798–806.
56. Armstrong DW 3rd, Rue JP, Wilckens JH, et al. Stress fracture injury in young military men and women. Bone 2004;35(3):806–16.
57. Giladi M, Ahronson Z, Stein M, et al. Unusual distribution and onset of stress fractures in soldiers. Clin Orthop Relat Res 1985;(192):142–6.
58. Greaney RB, Gerber FH, Laughlin RL, et al. Distribution and natural history of stress fractures in U.S. Marine recruits. Radiology 1983;146(2):339–46.
59. Green NE, Rogers RA, Lipscomb AB. Nonunions of stress fractures of the tibia. Am J Sports Med 1985;13(3):171–6.

60. Orava S, Hulkko A. Stress fracture of the mid-tibial shaft. Acta Orthop Scand 1984;55(1):35–7.

61. Kilcoyne KG, Dickens JF, Rue JP. Tibial stress fractures in an active duty population: long-term outcomes. J Surg Orthop Adv 2013;22(1):50–3.

62. Rettig AC, Shelbourne KD, McCarroll JR, et al. The natural history and treatment of delayed union stress fractures of the anterior cortex of the tibia. Am J Sports Med 1988;16(3):250–5.

63. Rue JP, Armstrong DW 3rd, Frassica FJ, et al. The effect of pulsed ultrasound in the treatment of tibial stress fractures. Orthopedics 2004;27(11):1192–5.

64. Borens O, Sen MK, Huang RC, et al. Anterior tension band plating for anterior tibial stress fractures in high-performance female athletes: a report of 4 cases. J Orthop Trauma 2006;20(6):425–30.

65. Chang PS, Harris RM. Intramedullary nailing for chronic tibial stress fractures. A review of five cases. Am J Sports Med 1996;24(5):688–92.

66. Kadel NJ, Teitz CC, Kronmal RA. Stress fractures in ballet dancers. Am J Sports Med 1992;20(4):445–9.

67. Carreira DA, Fox JA, Freedman KB, et al. Displaced nonunion patellar fracture following use of a patellar tendon autograft for ACL reconstruction: case report. J Knee Surg 2005;18(2):131–4.

68. Detterline AJ, Lattermann C, Bach BR Jr. Creation of transosseous patellar tunnels during extensor mechanism repair: technical note. J Knee Surg 2007;20(3): 249–50.

69. Gregory JM, Sherman SL, Mather R, et al. Patellar stress fracture after transosseous extensor mechanism repair: report of 3 cases. Am J Sports Med 2012; 40(7):1668–72.

70. Insall JN, Binazzi R, Soudry M, et al. Total knee arthroplasty. Clin Orthop Relat Res 1985;(192):13–22.

71. Devas MB. Stress fractures of the patella. J Bone Joint Surg Br 1960;42-B:71–4.

72. Hallel T, Amit S, Segal D. Fatigue fractures of tibial and femoral shaft in soldiers. Clin Orthop Relat Res 1976;(118):35–43.

73. Hopson CN, Perry DR. Stress fractures of the calcaneus in women marine recruits. Clin Orthop Relat Res 1977;(128):159–62.

74. Darby RE. Stress fractures of the os calcis. JAMA 1967;200(13):1183–4.

75. Sormaala MJ, Niva MH, Kiuru MJ, et al. Stress injuries of the calcaneus detected with magnetic resonance imaging in military recruits. J Bone Joint Surg Am 2006;88(10):2237–42.

76. Brukner P, Bradshaw C, Khan KM, et al. Stress fractures: a review of 180 cases. Clin J Sport Med 1996;6(2):85–9.

77. Bennell KL, Malcolm SA, Thomas SA, et al. The incidence and distribution of stress fractures in competitive track and field athletes. A twelve-month prospective study. Am J Sports Med 1996;24(2):211–7.

78. Khan KM, Brukner PD, Kearney C, et al. Tarsal navicular stress fracture in athletes. Sports Med 1994;17(1):65–76.

79. Khan KM, Fuller PJ, Brukner PD, et al. Outcome of conservative and surgical management of navicular stress fracture in athletes. Eighty-six cases proven with computerized tomography. Am J Sports Med 1992;20(6):657–66.

80. Saxena A, Fullem B. Navicular stress fractures: a prospective study on athletes. Foot Ankle Int 2006;27(11):917–21.

81. Saxena A, Fullem B, Hannaford D. Results of treatment of 22 navicular stress fractures and a new proposed radiographic classification system. J Foot Ankle Surg 2000;39(2):96–103.

82. Fitch KD, Blackwell JB, Gilmour WN. Operation for non-union of stress fracture of the tarsal navicular. J Bone Joint Surg Br 1989;71(1):105–10.

83. Torg JS, Moyer J, Gaughan JP, et al. Management of tarsal navicular stress fractures: conservative versus surgical treatment: a meta-analysis. Am J Sports Med 2010;38(5):1048–53.

84. Briethaupt M. Zur Pathologie Des Mensch Lichen Fusses [To the pathology of the humanfoot]. Med Zeitung 1855;(24):169–71, 175–7.

85. Bernstein A, Childers MA, et al. March fractures of the foot; care and management of 692 patients. Am J Surg 1946;71:355–62.

86. Boden BP, Osbahr DC, Jimenez C. Low-risk stress fractures. Am J Sports Med 2001;29(1):100–11.

87. Donahue SW, Sharkey NA. Strains in the metatarsals during the stance phase of gait: implications for stress fractures. J Bone Joint Surg Am 1999;81(9):1236–44.

88. Torg JS, Balduini FC, Zelko RR, et al. Fractures of the base of the fifth metatarsal distal to the tuberosity. Classification and guidelines for non-surgical and surgical management. J Bone Joint Surg Am 1984;66(2):209–14.

89. DeLee JC, Evans JP, Julian J. Stress fracture of the fifth metatarsal. Am J Sports Med 1983;11(5):349–53.

90. Steunebrink M, de Winter D, Tol JL. Bilateral stress fracture of the ulna in an adult weightlifter: a case report. Acta Orthop Belg 2008;74(6):851–5.

91. Kuo CL, Pan RY, Wu JL, et al. Stress fractures of forearm bones in military recruits of rifle drill training. J Trauma 2009;67(4):742–5.

92. Lin HH, Chang WH, Huang TF, et al. Bilateral stress fractures of the ulna in a young adolescent. J Pediatr Orthop B 2012;21(6):520–4.

93. Shelbourne KD, Fisher DA, Rettig AC, et al. Stress fractures of the medial malleolus. Am J Sports Med 1988;16(1):60–3.

94. Orava S, Karpakka J, Taimela S, et al. Stress fracture of the medial malleolus. J Bone Joint Surg Am 1995;77(3):362–5.

95. Van Hal ME, Keene JS, Lange TA, et al. Stress fractures of the great toe sesamoids. Am J Sports Med 1982;10(2):122–8.

96. DIPART (Vitamin D Individual Patient Analysis of Randomized Trials) Group. Patient level pooled analysis of 68 500 patients from seven major vitamin D fracture trials in US and Europe. BMJ 2010;340:b5463.

97. McCabe MP, Smyth MP, Richardson DR. Current concept review: vitamin D and stress fractures. Foot Ankle Int 2012;33(6):526–33.

98. Warden SJ, Hurst JA, Sanders MS, et al. Bone adaptation to a mechanical loading program significantly increases skeletal fatigue resistance. J Bone Miner Res 2005;20(5):809–16.

Seven Steps for Developing and Implementing a Preventive Training Program

Lessons Learned from JUMP-ACL and Beyond

Darin A. Padua, PhD[a],*, Barnett Frank, MA[b], Alex Donaldson, PhD[c],
Sarah de la Motte, PhD, MPH[d], Kenneth L. Cameron, PhD, MPH[e],
Anthony I. Beutler, MD[d], Lindsay J. DiStefano, PhD[f],
Stephen W. Marshall, PhD[g]

KEYWORDS

• Implementation • Injury prevention • Research framework • Program design
• Sports • Military

KEY POINTS

• The Translating Research into Injury Prevention Practice (TRIPP) framework describes 6 stages in injury prevention. This article provided details on implementing injury prevention movement training programs, with an emphasis on developing the injury prevention intervention (stage 3) and to describing the implementation context to inform implementation strategies (stage 5). This article addresses both the military and civilian settings.

• Establish administrative support for the preventive training program and develop an interdisciplinary implementation team of key stakeholders to identify implementation barriers and develop solutions to overcome these barriers before designing a preventive training program.

• Base preventive training programs on the best available evidence and engineer programs to address all identified implementation barriers.

Continued

[a] Department of Exercise and Sport Science, University of North Carolina, 204 Fetzer Hall, CB #8700, Chapel Hill, NC 27599-8700, USA; [b] Human Movement Science Curriculum, Department of Exercise and Sport Science, University of North Carolina, Chapel Hill, NC, USA; [c] Australian Centre for Research into Injury in Sport and its Prevention (ACRISP), Federation University Australia, SMB Campus, Ballarat, Victoria, Australia; [d] Consortium for Health and Military Performance, Uniformed Services University of the Health Sciences, Bethesda, MD, USA; [e] Keller Army Hospital, West Point, NY, USA; [f] Department of Kinesiology, University of Connecticut, Storrs, CT, USA; [g] Department of Epidemiology, University of North Carolina, Chapel Hill, NC, USA
* Corresponding author.
E-mail address: dpadua@email.unc.edu

Clin Sports Med 33 (2014) 615–632
http://dx.doi.org/10.1016/j.csm.2014.06.012
0278-5919/14/$ – see front matter © 2014 Elsevier Inc. All rights reserved.

Continued

- Establish a high level of competency and self-efficacy in the trainers who lead the exercises before going live with the preventive training program.
- Provide regular on-the-job coaching and feedback to trainers using positive reinforcement, simple and targeted suggestions of ways to improve, and quantitative measures of program fidelity.
- Reduce the frequency and quantity of on-the-job coaching and feedback to trainers as they meet objective criteria for high-fidelity implementation and performance of the program.

Musculoskeletal injuries place the greatest burden on military service members and the types of injuries sustained by military service members are similar to those commonly seen and treated in most sports medicine clinics elsewhere in this issue by Cameron and colleagues whether they are participating in military training activities or deployed in support of military operations such as Operation Enduring Freedom or Operation Iraqi Freedom.[1,2] Despite the growing understanding of the risk factors associated with the incidence of lower-extremity musculoskeletal injuries in military populations, implementing effective injury prevention programs within the context of the military has been challenging.[3] A major challenge to effective injury prevention practice is translating research outcomes into actions and programs that can be effectively implemented in real-world training settings.[4] Training programs designed to reduce the risk of these injuries in military training populations have shown promise[5]; however, the widespread implementation of these programs has not been realized. This article reviews critical steps in successfully developing and implementing injury prevention programs in military and civilian populations.[6]

Sports injury prevention research has often used a sequence of prevention model that outlines 4 steps needed to develop an evidence base about sports injuries and their causative factors.[7] However, this model does not take into consideration the need to translate research findings into practical, effective injury prevention interventions that can consistently be implemented in real-world settings.[4] This model does not consider the importance of implementation issues (such as ways to achieve widespread reach, adoption, compliance, and long-term maintenance) for prevention programs that have been proved to be effective. Descriptions and recommendations for implementing efficacious sports injury prevention programs in real-world settings are limited, although recent research suggests that investing in implementation planning can enhance intervention uptake in community sport.[8] The lack of attention to implementation issues in sports injury prevention research is a major factor limiting the ability to harness the potential of effective injury prevention. Deficiencies in the ability to translate research findings from controlled laboratory settings to the broader community and military greatly limits the public health impact of current prevention programs.[4,9–11]

Finch[4] identified the real-world implementation limitations of the sequence of prevention model, and proposed a 6-stage framework that expands on the original 4-step approach: the Translating Research into Injury Prevention Practice (TRIPP) framework. The TRIPP framework includes a focus on describing and assessing the intervention implementation context and the effectiveness of injury prevention programs in real-world settings.[4] However, the TRIPP framework does not provide specific guidance on the steps needed to develop and implement an evidence-based prevention program within the logistical constraints of a real-world setting. This article proposes 7 steps that can be used to operationalize stages 3 and 5 of the TRIPP framework and other models for behavioral health interventions (**Fig. 1**). These 7 steps are intended to guide the design and plan the implementation of an evidence-based preventive training program (PTP) within a real-world setting by identifying implementation barriers and associated solutions as a critical component of the process. This implementation is critical for injury prevention efforts in real-world settings because a one–size-fits-all approach is not always feasible across organizations and different high-risk populations (eg, military vs youth soccer).

The 7 steps for designing and planning the implementation of the PTP were informed by our experiences with the Joint Undertaking to Monitor and Prevent ACL Injury Study (JUMP-ACL study). The JUMP-ACL study began as a multisite prospective cohort study investigating biomechanical and neuromuscular risk factors for noncontact/indirect-contact ACL injury at the United States military, naval, and Air Force academies.[12] The second phase of JUMP-ACL focused on developing and implementing a PTP as part of a cluster randomized controlled trial at the United States Military Academy at West Point from 2010 to 2014. The PTP was delivered as a set of exercises performed as a dynamic warm-up before physical training. Our experiences during this phase of the JUMP-ACL study have led us to appreciate the importance of including additional steps within the TRIPP framework to optimize the translation of effective PTPs. By following these 7 steps during the PTP's design (TRIPP stage 3) and implementation planning (TRIPP stage 5) processes, we have been able to achieve high levels of compliance and implementation fidelity when implementing a PTP in a military setting.[13] We think that the lessons learned through this process also have utility in developing and implementing PTPs in youth sports and civilian populations at high risk for sports-related lower-extremity injuries.

ESTABLISH ADMINISTRATIVE SUPPORT

Assets and resources are typically focused on the mission of any organization and these behaviors reflect leadership priorities. Initiatives that do not have leadership support generally receive inadequate resources to support their initial and ongoing success. As a result, it is imperative to obtain leadership buy-in and support for injury prevention efforts and to ensure that an organization's leadership is committed to implementing any new intervention[14,15]; permission to implement should be negotiated before developing an intervention. If the PTP is not a leadership priority it is likely to have little chance of initial success and long-term sustainability within the target population, regardless of whether it is being implemented in a youth sports league or a military training environment.

To achieve permission to implement the PTP in the JUMP-ACL study, we met with key administrative leaders and stakeholders to brief them on the current science supporting PTPs and the potential benefits (ie, injury prevention and performance improvement) of implementing a PTP. We emphasized how these benefits were aligned with achieving the overall organizational mission and objectives; specifically, reducing the burden of lower-extremity musculoskeletal injuries, such as ACL tears and stress fractures, increasing force readiness, and limiting lost duty days caused by injury. A similar argument could be made to a youth soccer league board of directors that focuses on their concerns and goals (eg, player safety, improved performance, parent marketing) as an organization. As with the introduction of any innovation in an organization,[14] it is critical to show that the benefits of implementing a PTP are directly aligned with the overall mission and goals of the organization.

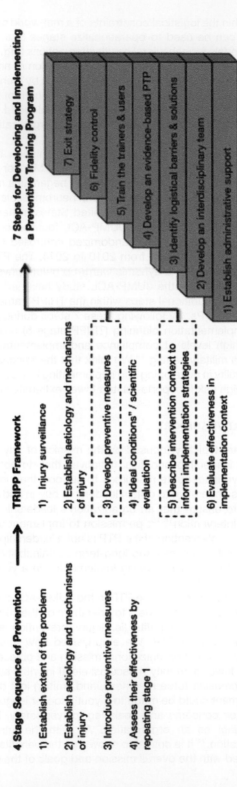

4 Stage Sequence of Prevention

1) Establish extent of the problem

2) Establish aetiology and mechanisms of injury

3) Introduce preventive measures

4) Assess their effectiveness by repeating stage 1

TRIPP Framework

1) Injury surveillance

2) Establish aetiology and mechanisms of injury

3) Develop preventive measures

4) "Ideal conditions" / scientific evaluation

5) Describe intervention context to inform implementation strategies

6) Evaluate effectiveness in implementation context

7 Steps for Developing and Implementing a Preventive Training Program

1) Establish administrative support

2) Develop an interdisciplinary team

3) Identify logistical barriers & solutions

4) Develop an evidence-based PTP

5) Train the trainers & users

6) Fidelity control

7) Exit strategy

Fig. 1. Seven steps for effective preventive training program (PTP) design and implementation: an evolution of sports injury prevention models.

Administrative leaders and stakeholders are more likely to implement new programs that are compatible with how they are evaluated for professional success.[16] Thus, when briefing administrative leaders and stakeholders we thought it was important to highlight how implementing a PTP could positively affect how they were evaluated for both individual and organizational success. For example, in a military training environment key metrics might include improvements in physical fitness as measured by the Army Physical Fitness Test or low attrition rates caused by injury. Aligning PTP outcomes with these organizational metrics can enhance buy-in and commitment from key stakeholders.

We highlighted the following points during our briefings to establish administrative support and buy-in for the PTP. First, we drew their attention to the negative outcomes associated with training-related injuries. We emphasized that such injuries are common, costly, result in significant time loss during training, reduce overall performance and military readiness, and ultimately decrease capacity to achieve organizational goals and mission-essential tasks. Second, we proactively addressed the common belief that implementing a PTP means that less time will be available for other training, thus detracting from organizational goals and success. To do this we highlighted previous research showing that PTPs can be completed in short time periods[17] and are effective in decreasing musculoskeletal injury rates[17–19] and improving athletic performance.[17,20,21] We thought it was important to emphasize how implementing a PTP does not detract from the organization's goals but reduces overall costs while simultaneously improving performance. These benefits may help improve organizational efficiency and augment the positive effects of other training measures to achieve organizational success.

Another common barrier for achieving permission to implement can be an organization's belief that the program that is in place is already achieving the desired outcome. To overcome this barrier in the JUMP-ACL study we provided information to the administrative leadership and key stakeholders. We emphasized that the existing warm-up program did not incorporate evidence-based exercises shown to improve biomechanics associated with injury risk and mechanisms, reduce injury rates, and improve athletic performance measures. Thus, we highlighted the advantage of what was being proposed compared with the current practice[15] and the benefits of refining and optimizing what was already in place and working together to design and implement an evidence-based PTP. This process allowed us to collaborate with the administrative leaders and stakeholders in developing a PTP that was aligned with their organizational goals and that would fit within the context of existing schedules and programs. This type of collaborative program design may help establish trust with the organization and ultimately achieve permission to implement. This approach is also likely to foster support for long-term sustainability following the initial implementation cycle, which is important when developing an exit strategy, as outlined later.

DEVELOP AN INTERDISCIPLINARY IMPLEMENTATION TEAM

Having obtained administrative support for program implementation, we developed an interdisciplinary implementation team to assist with developing the PTP and its associated implementation strategy, which is in line with key steps in a range of implementation planning frameworks and processes described in the literature.[14,22] We involved key stakeholders to ensure that the PTP we developed was both evidence based and context specific. Key stakeholders may include program implementers (those involved in program development and operations), partners (those who actively support the program), participants (those served or affected by the program), and decision makers (those in a position to do or decide something about the program). In the context of implementing a PTP, key stakeholders may include program designers, trainers, end users (eg, noncommissioned officers, coaches), health care providers, and administrators. It may also be important to engage potential critics or adversaries of the program to avoid potential barriers during implementation. In working with community-based programs it is also probably important to include athletes, parents, coaches, and other stakeholders who may have a vested interest in the PTP within the target population.

The primary role of the interdisciplinary implementation team was to identify and suggest possible solutions for all potential logistical issues that could negatively influence the fidelity, compliance, and long-term adoption of the PTP. It was also important to attempt to limit the impact of any injury prevention efforts on activities that organizational leaders deemed critical to their primary mission (training military officers). This goal was accomplished by the interdisciplinary team through working closely with leaders and key stake holders to identify the proper timing and sequence for PTP delivery around mission essential activities. We achieved a comprehensive, multiperspective view of potential logistical barriers to implementation through our discussions. Recommendations for exercise inclusion were solicited from these key stakeholders to ensure that the PTP was not only focused on injury prevention but also on improving physical performance in areas that were important to the organization. For example, push-up performance is important for the military and the push-up is also a good exercise to work on core stability when performed correctly, so this exercise was included in our PTP to satisfy the shared goals of the organization and program planners.

IDENTIFY LOGISTICAL BARRIERS AND SOLUTIONS

We grouped the identified implementation barriers into 4 main categories: time, personnel, environment, and organization.

Time

- Time of day the PTP would be performed
- Duration of each PTP session
- Frequency with which the PTP would be performed each week
- Opportunity costs for using training time for PTP

Personnel

- Experience and expertise of those leading the PTP
- Baseline movement quality of those performing the PTP
- Previous experience in performing injury prevention exercises of those performing the PTP

Environment

- Location/setting in which the PTP will be performed
- Equipment available when performing the PTP

Organization

- Organizational goals and metrics of success
- Current warm-up endorsed by the organization

Once identified, in partnership with the interdisciplinary implementation team we mapped a set of potential solutions to address each of the implementation barriers. In line with the concept of developing health behavior change interventions with the application in mind,[23] the solutions were then incorporated into the design of the evidence-based PTP and integrated into the overall implementation strategy. An example of the solutions map for the implementation barriers is provided in **Table 1**.

Table 1
Map of logistical implementation barriers and associated solutions

PTP Design	Identified Implementation Barrier	Solution
Total program duration	5 wk to implement the PTP	Identify key PTP goals that could be attained in 6 wk and design PTP accordingly
Session duration	12 min to complete PTP each training session	Determine exercises that can achieve identified PTP goals (discussed earlier) and be performed and mastered within the allocated time
	Additional time may be available to complete the PTP on certain days because of overall training schedule	If individuals have not mastered exercises, then repeat those exercises If time permits, repeat more demanding exercises
Location	PTP will be performed in different locations on a regular basis	Visit each location in which PTP will be performed and ensure that exercises can be performed in that location
	PTP will be performed in small areas with individuals tightly grouped together	Select PTP exercises that can be performed in a stationary location
Organization's goals	Pass physical fitness test at end of training period	Show that the PTP will not detract from passing physical fitness test, and may enhance performance and ability to pass physical fitness test
	Develop fundamental skills	Show that the time to complete the PTP will not infringe on other training goals and will accomplish the goal to warm up before other physical training Show how mastering the PTP exercises develops fundamental motor skills that may improve ability to master other fundamental skills
	Develop leadership skills	Show that PTP can provide opportunities for leadership development with those leading the exercises and by providing feedback to others on PTP quality
Success metrics	40 push-ups in 2 min 100 sit-ups in 2 min 2.4-km (1.5-mile) run in 10 min	Ensure that administrators, implementers, and users see how the selected PTP exercises contribute to meeting these success metrics. Show that the program has face validity
Equipment	No available equipment to use with PTP implementation	Select PTP exercises that do not require use of additional equipment

DEVELOP AN EVIDENCE-BASED AND CONTEXT-APPROPRIATE PTP

The specific PTP exercises were selected after a systematic review of the existing literature to identify those exercises previously used in successful PTPs while considering the previously identified context-specific implementation barriers. Exercises that were evidence-based, would best meet the needs of the organization, and would address the implementation barriers were selected for inclusion in the PTP. As noted earlier, we also worked with the interdisciplinary team and key stakeholders to select exercises that would also support and enhance military physical performance. The outcome of this process was the Dynamic Integrated Movement Efficiency (DIME) PTP (**Fig. 2**). The DIME PTP represents an evidence-based PTP that provides solutions for the problem of lower-extremity injuries within the organization. Furthermore, the DIME PTP was designed to be performed within the previously identified logistical constraints and align with organizational goals for success.

The specific exercises included in the DIME PTP were only finalized after achieving administrative support, establishing an interdisciplinary team, and identifying appropriate solutions to all implementation barriers. Implementation of injury prevention programs traditionally begins with trying to convince an organization that they should adopt a preestablished set of exercises. This approach often results in suboptimal levels of compliance and long-term maintenance.[8,24,25] This traditional approach is not based on a collaborative process between administrative leaders, key stakeholders, and those seeking to develop and implement the PTP. Often this is a lost opportunity to develop a level of trust between all parties and ensure that the mutual goals of all key stakeholders are addressed during the development and implementation of the PTP. In addition, the preestablished set of exercises may not fit the implementation context or take the implementation barriers of the organization and setting into account. Although it is important to have a general idea for the specific evidence-based exercises to be included in the PTP, the content of the PTP should not be finalized until going through the initial 3 steps, thus ensuring that the program is collaboratively designed, meets the organization's needs, and can be implemented within the identified logistical constraints. These steps are critical to facilitate buy-in and support for the program among key stakeholders and end users, and are likely to enhance long-term sustainability following the initial implementation cycle.

TRAIN THE TRAINERS AND USERS

After working with key stakeholders to develop the DIME PTP, we then developed educational strategies and support materials to train those who would be leading the program (trainers) and delivering it to the end users. To address one of the acknowledged key drivers of implementation success,[9] the goal was to develop high levels of competency and self-efficacy among the trainers who would be leading the DIME PTP. In addition, we sought to achieve buy-in from the trainers by highlighting that the organization supported the implementation of the DIME PTP and that it was aligned with organizational goals for success. We focused our train-the-trainer process on 5 areas: effectiveness, alignment, knowledge, self-efficacy, and feedback.

A 2-hour educational workshop was held a month before implementing the DIME PTP. The workshop was divided into lecture and hands-on application components. During the lecture we addressed the areas of effectiveness, alignment, and knowledge to instill a positive attitude for performing the DIME exercises in the trainers. Effectiveness was addressed by highlighting the positive outcomes associated with implementing the PTP, such as reduced injury rates,[17–19] reduced organizational costs,[26] and improved organizational performance.[27] We also emphasized how the DIME

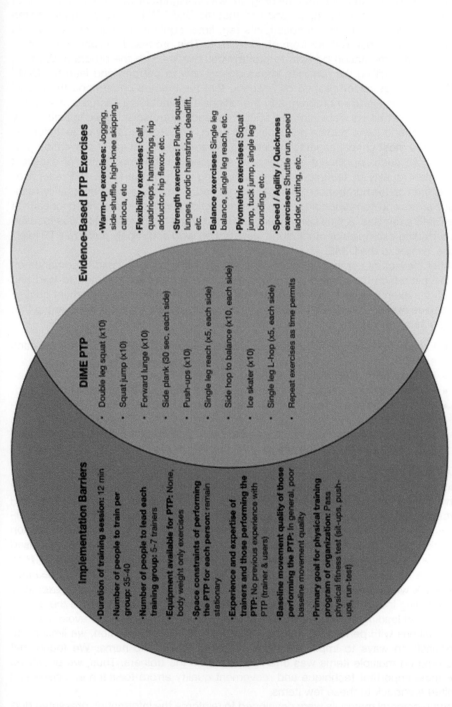

Implementation Barriers

- Duration of training session: 12 min
- Number of people to train per group: 35-40
- Number of people to lead each training group: 5-7 trainers
- Equipment available for PTP: None, body weight only exercises
- Space constraints of performing the PTP for each person: remain stationary
- Experience and expertise of trainers and those performing the PTP: No previous experience with PTP (trainer & users)
- Baseline movement quality of those performing the PTP: In general, poor baseline movement quality
- Primary goal for physical training program of organization: Pass physical fitness test (sit-ups, push-ups, run-test)

DIME PTP

- Double leg squat (x10)
- Squat jump (x10)
- Forward lunge (x10)
- Side plank (30 sec, each side)
- Push-ups (x10)
- Single leg reach (x5, each side)
- Side hop to balance (x10, each side)
- Ice skater (x10)
- Single leg L-hop (x5, each side)
- Repeat exercises as time permits

Evidence-Based PTP Exercises

- Warm-up exercises: Jogging, side-shuffle, high-knee skipping, carioca, etc
- Flexibility exercises: Calf, quadriceps, hamstrings, hip adductor, hip flexor, etc.
- Strength exercises: Plank, squat, lunges, nordic hamstring, deadlift, etc.
- Balance exercises: Single leg balance, single leg reach, etc.
- Plyometric exercises: Squat jump, tuck jump, single leg bounding, etc.
- Speed / Agility / Quickness exercises: Shuttle run, speed ladder, cutting, etc.

Fig. 2. Development of the DIME PTP using a solutions-oriented process to address implementation barriers using evidence-based exercises for injury prevention.

PTP was designed by an interdisciplinary team, including their organizational leaders and stakeholders, ensuring that the program was in alignment with the overall goals of the organization. In addition, we showed that the DIME PTP could be implemented within the identified logistical constraints (eg, time, equipment, location) and would enhance, rather than detract from other training. This process highlighted that there were no implementation barriers to prohibit compliance with the program. We then focused on instilling the requisite knowledge of how to perform and lead the DIME PTP, which was accomplished by ensuring that the trainers understood the overall purpose of the exercise program and the rationale for including each exercise in the program. The trainers were informed about how each exercise achieved specific injury prevention and performance enhancement goals. Movement quality or technique is one of the most critical aspects influencing the success of an injury prevention program.[28] As such, significant emphasis was placed on the importance of excellent movement quality or technique when performing each of the DIME PTP exercises rather than on the number of repetitions completed. Common movement quality/technique errors and corresponding corrective instructions were also described for each of the DIME exercises. A final component of developing a positive attitude was focused on providing examples of other high-level athletes who commonly perform PTP exercises, similar to the DIME.

After the lecture component of the educational workshop, we conducted hands-on training in which the trainers performed each of the exercises, learned to lead and teach the exercises, and practiced providing feedback to correct movement quality/technique errors. During the hands-on training process we focused on ensuring that the trainers were able to:

- Explain the rationale (injury prevention and performance enhancement) for each exercise
- Perform each exercise with proper technique
- Identify technique errors and poor movement quality during each exercise
- Provide general and targeted instructional cues to improve technique and movement quality
- Modify the difficulty level of each exercise to ensure that proper technique and movement quality was achieved

After conducting several hands-on train-the-trainer sessions, strategies to better engage with the trainers and achieve higher levels of buy-in and self-efficacy were developed. First, we identified that it was important to always provide positive reinforcement when educating trainers about the rationale and how to perform the exercises. Most trainers had no experience with performing or leading injury prevention exercises and had minimal expertise in assessing movement quality. Thus, we used positive reinforcement when coaching the trainers on their leading of the PTP to keep the trainers committed to the DIME PTP. Second, we avoided using negative feedback when correcting the trainers on how they were performing the exercises or providing instructions to others. Instead we identified ways to improve the performance and leading of the exercises by the trainer, which was done to avoid negative associations with performing and leading the DIME PTP. In addition, we limited our feedback on ways to improve to only a few (2–3) specific items. We found that focusing on multiple items was often confusing to the trainers. Thus, we prioritized the most important technique and movement quality errors for each exercises and limited feedback to these few items.

Supplemental materials were developed to reinforce the information presented during the educational workshop. This trainers' toolkit included a detailed handbook describing each DIME PTP exercise, a laminated 22 × 28 cm (8.5 × 11 inch) clipboard sheet with an overview of each exercise (**Fig. 3**). The clipboard sheet also included reminders of common errors and instructional cues to provide when leading the DIME PTP exercises. In addition, trainers were given details of a Web site (http://dimeinjuryprevention.weebly.com/) containing videos of:

- Examples of correct performance of each of the DIME PTP exercises
- Examples of common exercise technique errors and corresponding instructional cues
- Quizzes to identify those performing exercises with good and poor technique
- Discussions of real-world applications of DIME PTP exercises
- Supporting research for implementing the DIME PTP

The purpose of the trainers' toolkit was to further improve the trainers' perceived control and self-efficacy for implementing the DIME PTP.

Providing adequate training and support materials to those who will be implementing the PTP is critical. We solicited input from the trainers during the initial development and pilot testing of the DIME and modified or added support materials that they suggested would enhance their confidence and ability to model, teach, and provide feedback on the PTP exercises. The overall goal was to establish the background knowledge and confidence to implement the program, ensure that all trainers could perform all exercises, and to ensure that they could identify and correct critical movement errors. To ensure that this was achieved we also implemented strategies to monitor fidelity control and provide feedback to trainers during the implementation process.

FIDELITY CONTROL

The DIME PTP was implemented 3 to 5-times per week over a 5-week training period (17 total training sessions). In order to provide on-the-job coaching and performance assessment[29] we developed a scoring rubric to evaluate the fidelity of implementation of the DIME PTP (**Fig. 4**). During each training session we evaluated the leadership abilities of the trainers as they led their groups through the DIME PTP exercises. We also evaluated how well the group performed each exercise and the ability of each trainer to provide appropriate instructional cues. Leadership, exercise execution, and overall scores were then developed based on the evaluation rubric. At the end of each training session we reviewed scores with the trainer and provided feedback on a few key ways to improve for the next training session. This information was also translated to key members of the leadership team during the intervention cycle.

We thought it important to establish positive associations with leading and performing the exercises to achieve long-term adoption and compliance with the DIME PTP. Thus, many of the lessons learned during the initial pilot train-the-trainer sessions were applied when providing on-the-job coaching and feedback to the trainers after each training session (eg, positive reinforcement, ways to improve), because we did not want to facilitate any negative associations. In the future, it may be important to emphasize to the end user that after performing the DIME exercises they are now warmed up and ready the remainder of their training program. This emphasis may help to establish a sense of achievement and reward when completing a PTP, thus helping to facilitate the desire to continue to perform the exercises in the future.

EXIT STRATEGY

Given the existing logistical constraints of a military training environment, we provided support for the implementation of the DIME PTP over a 5-week training period.

USMA Dynamic Integrated Movement Enhancement

Exercise	Description	Coaching Cues
1. Double Leg Squat 	**Starting position**: Feet shoulder width apart, hands on hip bones. **Directions**: Squat down slowly, sending hips back as if sitting in a chair. Knees bend to 90 degrees. Return to standing. Back stays flat throughout. **Cadence: Slow** (♩= 40) **Reps: 10**	• "Knees over toes" • "Keep knees from going past toes" • "Toes straight ahead" • "Sit back" • "Feet shoulder width apart"
2. Squat Jump 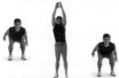	**Starting position**: Squat position, arms in ready position in front. **Directions**: Jump up for maximum height and return to start position. Land softly toe to heel. Control the landing by bending at the hips, knees and ankles. **Cadence:Moderate** (♩= 60) **Reps: 5, rest, 5**	• "Land *softly* toe to heel" • "Bend at the hips, knees, and ankles" • "Knees over toes" • "Toes straight ahead" • "Jump for maximum height"

Key Points to Emphasize for EVERY Exercise!

  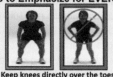 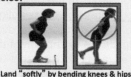

Keep toes pointing straight ahead   Keep knees directly over the toes   Land "softly" by bending knees & hips

Exercise	Description	Coaching Cues
3. Forward Lunge 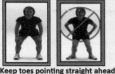	**Starting position**: Feet hip-distance apart, hands on hips. **Directions**: Take a long step forward with left foot and slowly lower back knee toward ground. Push with front leg to return to standing. Alternate legs. **Cadence: Slow** (♩= 40) **Reps: 10**	• "Knees over toes" • "Keep knees behind toes" • "Bend both knees to 90" • "Keep torso upright"
4. Side Plank 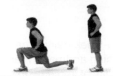	**Starting position:** Side lying on left side, elbow under shoulder, feet stacked. **Directions:** Lift your hips, bringing them in a straight line with shoulder & feet. Brace abs & glutes. Hold 30 sec, maintaining straight line head to spine. **Cadence: Stationary 30 count each side**	• "Straight line, head to toes" • "Keep hips perpendicular with ground" • "Brace abs & squeeze your glutes" • "Elbow directly under shoulder"
5. Push-Up 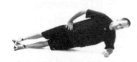 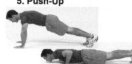	**Starting position**: Front leaning rest. **Directions**: Maintain a flat back and brace the abs. Lower body to ground, keeping elbows in. Push up to starting position. **Cadence: Moderate Reps: 10**	• "Keep back flat, don't sag" • "Keep abs braced" • "Hands directly under shoulders" • "Don't lock elbows"

Fig. 3. Clipboard sheets provided as supplemental educational materials to facilitate high-fidelity implementation of the DIME PTP by trainers. (*Courtesy of* JUMP-ACL Research Team, All rights reserved, 2012.)

Time-based completion of PTPs may not be ideal for achieving success and an alternative approach based on achieving predefined goals may be more desirable if it fits within the implementation context. Objective criteria for achieving high-fidelity implementation should be established by the interdisciplinary implementation team during step 2, and this can be evaluated using a fidelity score, as previously described. Once predefined levels of high-fidelity implementation have been achieved it may be

USMA Dynamic Integrated Movement Enhancement

Exercise	Description	Coaching Cues
6. Single Leg Reach 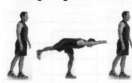	**Starting position:** Standing on left leg with knee slightly bent. **Directions:** Extend arms by ears and tip forward at the hips, extending right leg to the rear. Keep hips level. Return to standing. Left leg stays slightly bent. **Cadence: Slow** (♩= 40) **Reps: 5 each side**	• "Hips level" • "Keep back flat" • "Keep your balance" • "Tip forward at the hip" • "Rear leg reaches back"
7. Side Hop to Balance 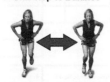	**Starting position:** Left foot with knee bent, hands on hips. **Directions:** Hop sideways, as if over a hurdle, and land on opposite foot. Bend at hips, knees and ankles. Hold balance for 2 seconds. Hop back to other side & repeat. **Cadence: Slow** (♩= 40) **Reps: 10, rest, 10**	• "Land *softly* toe to heel" • "Keep center of gravity low" • "Knees over toes" • "Toes straight ahead" • "Keep your balance"

Key Points to Emphasize for EVERY Exercise!

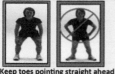 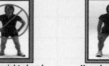 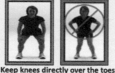   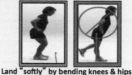

Keep toes pointing straight ahead	Keep knees directly over the toes	Land "softly" by bending knees & hips

Exercise	Description	Coaching Cues
8. Ice Skater 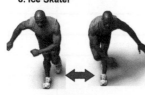	**Starting position:** Left leg with knee bent, ready position. **Directions:** Hop sideways and land softly on the opposite foot, bending at hips, knees, and ankles. Hop immediately back to starting foot. Control the landing, maintain balance & stay low. **Cadence: Moderate** (♩= 60) **Reps: 10**	• "Hop and land *softly*" • "Keep center of gravity low" • "Knees over toes" • "Explode back to other side"
9. "L" Hop 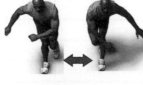 2, 4 └→ 3 │ 1	**Starting position:** Left foot with knee bent, hands on hips **Directions:** Hop forward and land softly on left foot, bending at hips, knees, & ankles. Hop quickly back to start position. Hop to the left & back to start. Repeat for 5 reps. Repeat on the right leg in the opposite direction (forward, backward, right, back to start). **Cadence: Slow** (♩= 40) **Reps: 5 each side**	• "Hop and land *softly* • "Bend hips, knees, & ankles" • "Keep your chest over your foot" • "Get off the ground when hopping"

Fig. 3. (*continued*)

appropriate to scale back the level of support. For example, transitioning from daily on-the-job coaching and feedback to 2 to 3 times per week may be appropriate once high-fidelity implementation is achieved. Assuming that implementation fidelity remains high, further reducing the level of support to random observations can occur over time. However, if implementation fidelity decreases, then it may be appropriate to increase monitoring frequency and provide additional on-the-job coaching and feedback. The key is to have predefined objective criteria for the withdrawal of support that are based on program fidelity, not simply time if possible.

Initials of Person Completing this Form: [   ][   ][   ]

DIME CHECKLIST

Company	B / D / F / H	Time Plt Arrived [ ]	(hhmm)
Platoon	1 / 2 / 3 / 4	Time Exercises Started [ ]	(hhmm)
Date	[/ /]	Time Exercises Stopped [ ]	(hhmm)

LEADERSHIP	1	2	3	4	5	
A. Platoon set in correct formation (expanded spacing)						
B. All Instructors correctly demonstrate exercises						
C. All Instructors maintain good cadence (slower is better)						
D. Cadre mobile in platoon (without prompting)						
E. Cadre provide targeted and general coaching cues (without prompting)						

Sum of Scores for A to E [   ]

Leadership Score (number above multiplied by 2) [   ]

MOVEMENT	Things to improve	Cadet Performance	Cadre Corrections	sum of Performance and Corrections
1. Double Leg Squat	sit back / toes straight ahead / knees over toes / keep hips level	1 2 3 4 5	1 2 3 4 5	
2. Squat Jump	jump as high as you can / land softly / toes straight ahead / knees over toes	1 2 3 4 5	1 2 3 4 5	
3. Forward Lunge	step out far enough / toes straight ahead / knees over toes / keep torso upright	1 2 3 4 5	1 2 3 4 5	
4. Side Plank	elbow directly under shoulder / don't sag or twist / keep hips perpendicular to the ground / keep abs tight	1 2 3 4 5	1 2 3 4 5	
5. Push-up	hands directly under shoulders / keep back flat / keep abs tight / elbows straighten but do not lock	1 2 3 4 5	1 2 3 4 5	
6. Single Leg Reach	tip forward at the hip / rear leg reaches back / keep back flat / hips level / keep your balance	1 2 3 4 5	1 2 3 4 5	
7. Side Hop to Balance	land softly / knees over toes / toes straight ahead / don't let knee wobble / hold balance for 2 sec	1 2 3 4 5	1 2 3 4 5	
8. Ice Skater	land softly / keep center of gravity low / knees over toes / toes straight ahead	1 2 3 4 5	1 2 3 4 5	
9. "L" Hop	land softly / bend hips, knees, and ankles / land toe to heel / knee in line with toes / keep your balance	1 2 3 4 5	1 2 3 4 5	
10. General Impression		1 2 3 4 5	1 2 3 4 5	

Sum of Scores for 1-10 [   ]

Movement Score (number above divided by 2) [   ]

OBSERVATIONS

V6 6/1/2012

Fig. 4. Scoring rubric to evaluate fidelity of DIME PTP implementation. CBT, cadet basic training; Plt, platoon.

Following the training period the interdisciplinary implementation team met to discuss ways to refine the DIME PTP design and implementation strategies in the future. All members of the interdisciplinary implementation team were asked to provide feedback on ways to address potential barriers for long-term adoption across all administrative levels. To ensure long-term adoption and PTP sustainability we developed strategies for addressing each of the issues raised and presented these solutions to the team at a later date and sought their feedback and consultation, which allowed us to continue the collaborative process of refining and implementing the DIME PTP. It also allowed us to provide materials and resources that the end users deemed important to support ongoing sustainability for the program.

SCORING GUIDE		
"CORE" CUES	▪"TOES STRAIGHT AHEAD"	
FOR EVERY	▪"KNEES OVER TOES"	
EXERCISE	▪"LAND SOFTLY -- By Bending Knees & Hips"	

Additional Cues & Corrections	1. Double Leg Squat	▪"Sit Back - Keep Heels on Ground" ▪"Keep Knees from going past Toes"	
	2. Squat Jump	▪"Jump as High as You Can" ▪"Land *Softly* -- Toe to Heel"	▪"Knees over Toes"
	3. Forward Lunge	▪"Keep Torso upright" ▪"Step Out far enough to keep Knees from going past Toes"	▪"Knees over Toes"
	4. Side Plank	▪"Keep Abs Tight" ▪"Keep Back Flat -- Don't Sag or Twist!"	▪"Elbows Directly under Shoulders"
	5. Push-up	▪"Keep Abs Tight" ▪"Keep Back Flat -- Don't Sag!"	
	6. Single Leg Reach	▪"Keep Back Flat" ▪"Keep Hips Level"	
	7. Side Hop to Balance	▪"Land Toe to Heel" ▪"Hop and Land *Softly* with Bent Knees, Hips, and Trunk"	
	8. Ice Skater	▪"Hop and Land *Softly* with Bent Knees, Hips, and Trunk" ▪"Keep Center of Gravity low"	▪"Be Fluid"
	9. "L" Hop	▪"Hop and Land *Softly* with Bent Knees, Hips, and Trunk" ▪"Keep Knees in Line With Toes" ▪"Bend Hips, Knees, and Ankles"	
	General Impression	*Effort in 1-on-1 Coaching, AARs w/- DIME team, etc.*	

LEADERSHIP RUBRIC
A. PLATOON FORMATION -- Set up with arms FULLY extended plus 2 inches, equipment grounded safely at front right, instructors reset platoon as needed
5=Cadets are able to perform ALL exercises correctly and safely
4=Formation is correct at the beginning, cadre correct spacing AFTER problems
3=Formation is correct at beginning but cadre do not fix collapsing formation
2=Cadets are unable to perform 2 or more exercises correctly due to formation
1=Formation is not set properly at beginning and cadre make no corrections
B. CORRECTLY DEMONSTRATES EXERCISES -- per CBT Physical Program Manual/Clipboard Sheet
5=all 9 exercises described clearly in audible voice and demonstrated correctly
4=8 of 9 exercises demonstrated correctly, directions are mostly clear
3=average demonstrations and descriptions
2=3 or more exercises demonstrated poorly, cadets are not sure what to do
1=poor demonstrations and inaudible or unclear directions
C. MAINTAIN GOOD CADENCE: -- per CBT Physical Program Manual/Clipboard Sheet
5=all exercises are demonstrated AND led with correct and consistent cadence
4=1 exercise performed too quickly or with an inconsistent cadence
3=2 exercises performed too quickly or with an inconsistent cadence
2=3 or more exercises performed too quickly
1=Most exercises performed too quickly or with an inconsistent cadence
D. CADRE MOBILE IN PLT -- Move throughout formation to observe ALL cadets on EVERY exercise
5=ALL Cadre are constantly observing and moving toward cadets with many errors
4=ALL Cadre move throughout the formation
3=Cadre move around the outside of the formation
2=Some cadre move around the formation
1=Most cadre move infrequently or watch from the back of the formation
E. CONSTANTLY PROVIDE TARGETED CUES -- Cadre constantly state cues, appropriate to specific cadet errors
5=Coaching cues used frequently and appropriately targeted to specific cadet errors
4=Some cadre frequently use targeted cues for specific errors and all cadre give appropriate cues for each exercise
3=Cadre provide cues but NOT targeted to specific cadet errors
2=Some cadre provide coaching cues to entire platoon
1=A few cadre use cues sporadically or inappropriately

MOVEMENT RUBRIC
CADET PERFORMANCE
5=Close to 100% of the cadets are performing to standard, others are making minor errors
4=75% are performing to standard, other making some errors
3=50% are performing to standard, others are making frequent errors
2=Less than 50% are performing to standard, others make frequent errors or cannot perform the exercise
1=The majority of cadets (>75%) are performing the exercise incorrectly or cannot perform the exercise
CADRE CORRECTIONS
5=Coaching cues used frequently and appropriately targeted to specific cadet errors
4=Some cadre frequently use targeted cues for specific errors and all cadre give appropriate cues for each exercise
3=Cadre provide cues but NOT targeted to specific cadet errors
2=Some cadre provide coaching cues to entire platoon
1=A few cadre use cues sporadically or inappropriately

Fig. 4. *(continued)*

The exit strategy should also consider ways to embed the implementation strategies (eg, educational workshop, hands-on training, on-the-job coaching, and feedback) into the systems of the organization. Future high-fidelity implementation of the PTP requires continued delivery of these implementation strategies, thus these strategies need to become part of the organizations normal operating procedures. Data that the organization routinely collects (eg, fitness test scores, injury surveillance data) may be used to support the ongoing implementation (maintenance) of the PTP. For example, highlighting positive associations between PTP implementation with fitness test scores and injury rate reductions may strengthen the organization's long-term commitment to implementing the PTP (maintenance).

SUMMARY

Our experience implementing the DIME PTP in a real-world military training environment led to the development of the 7 steps for PTP design and implementation planning that can be used to operationalize stages 3 and 5 of the TRIPP framework and other models for implementing behavioral health interventions. Perhaps the most important lesson learned was the significance of working with an interdisciplinary implementation team to consider the intervention implementation context and identify implementation barriers with associated solutions before designing the final version of the PTP. To date, most of the research on sport injury prevention programs has focused solely on the content of the program (ie, the specific exercise selection and program duration) without considering the context in which the program is to be implemented by other key stakeholders including the program trainers, coaches, and end users.

Our experience suggests that to achieve optimal implementation compliance and long-term adoption (maintenance) and sustainability administrative support must first be developed within the organization for which the PTP is intended. After administrative support is established, it is imperative that an interdisciplinary implementation team be developed comprising key stakeholders from multiple levels within the target organization. Development of an interdisciplinary implementation team will ensure the most effective and efficient identification of barriers before implementation of the PTP, which may otherwise be ignored if stakeholders from multiple sectors of the intervention context are not involved in the planning process. Potential program critics should also be consulted during the process to identify potential barriers. Identifying barriers to implementation before PTP implementation facilitates development of an evidence-based and context-appropriate PTP that has a greater probability of widespread adoption, high-level implementation compliance, maintenance, and sustainability within the target organization.

Once the PTP has been designed to circumvent implementation barriers, the program is ready for implementation within the target organization, and leaders can be trained to implement the program effectively. It is vital that the implementation team establishes a high level of competence and self-efficacy in the trainers to ensure that they are comfortable instructing individuals how to perform the exercises successfully as intended before initiating the PTP. Trainers should also consider themselves to be competent in exercise error identification and correction. As trainers develop a high level of competence and self-efficacy they can be transitioned into receiving on-the-job coaching and feedback over a decreasing schedule. However, the feedback schedule should only be decreased as the organization meets objective checkpoints for high-fidelity implementation and performance of the PTP. Once objective high-fidelity implementation of the PTP is achieved, the implementation team can begin to withdraw from the target organization with a planned exit strategy that facilitates long-term sustainability and maintenance of the PTP. Integrating these 7 steps as part of the PTP design and implementation strategy can enhance the effectiveness and sustainability of an injury prevention program in real-world settings.

REFERENCES

1. Hauret K, Taylor B, Clemmons N, et al. Frequency and causes of nonbattle injuries air evacuated from operations Iraqi freedom and enduring freedom, US Army, 2001–2006. Am J Prev Med 2010;8:S94–107.
2. Jones B, Knapik J. Physical training and exercise-related injuries. Surveillance, research and injury prevention in military populations. Sports Med 1999;27: 111–25.
3. Finestone A, Milgrom C. How stress fracture incidence was lowered in the Israeli army: a 25-yr struggle. Med Sci Sports Exerc 2008;40:S623–9.
4. Finch C. A new framework for research leading to sports injury prevention. J Sci Med Sport 2006;9:3–9.
5. Bullock S, Jones B, Gilchrist J, et al. Prevention of physical training-related injuries recommendations for the military and other active populations based on expedited systematic reviews. Am J Prev Med 2010;38:S156–81.
6. Gielen A, McDonald E, Gary T, et al. Using the PRECEDE-PROCEDE model to apply health behavior theories. In: Glanz K, Rimer B, Viswanath K, editors. Health behavior and health education: theory, research, and practice. 4th edition. San Francisco: Jossey-Bass; 2008. p. 407–29.
7. van Mechelen W, Hlobil H, Kemper H. Incidence, severity, aetiology, and prevention of sports injuries. A review of concepts. Sports Med 1992;14:82–99.
8. Poulos R, Donaldson A. Improving the diffusion of safety initiatives in community sport. J Sci Med Sport 2014. [Epub ahead of print].
9. Donaldson A, Finch C. Applying implementation science to sports injury prevention. Br J Sports Med 2013;47:473–5.
10. Sugimoto D, Myer G, McKeon J, et al. Evaluation of the effectiveness of neuromuscular training to reduce anterior cruciate ligament injury in female athletes: a critical review of relative risk reduction and numbers-needed-to-treat analyses. Br J Sports Med 2012;46:979–88.
11. Hanson D, Allegrante JA, Sleet D, et al. Research alone is not sufficient to prevent sports injury. Br J Sports Med 2014;48(8):682–4.
12. Padua D. Executing a collaborative prospective risk-factor study: findings, successes, and challenges. J Athl Train 2010;45:519–21.
13. Beutler A, de la Motte S, Distefano L, et al. Can a 10-minute injury prevention program decrease injuries in military cadets? A JUMP-ACL study. In: abstracts from American Medical Society for sports medicine 22nd annual meeting. San Diego: 2013. Clin J Sport Med 2013;23:123–56.
14. Meyers D, Durlak J, Wandersman A. The quality implementation framework: a synthesis of critical steps in the implementation process. Am J Community Psychol 2012;50:462–80.
15. Damschroder L, Aron D, Keith R, et al. Fostering implementation of health services research findings into practice: a consolidated framework for advancing implementation science. Implement Sci 2009;4:50.
16. Greenhalgh T, Robert G, Macfarlane F, et al. Diffusion of innovations in service organizations: systematic review and recommendations. Milbank Q 2004;82: 581–629.
17. Sadoghi P, von Keudell A, Vavken P. Effectiveness of anterior cruciate ligament injury prevention training programs. Am J Bone Joint Surg 2012;94:769–76.
18. LaBella C, Huxford M, Grissom J, et al. Effect of neuromuscular warm-up on injuries in female soccer and basketball athletes in urban public high schools: cluster randomized controlled trial. Arch Pediatr Adolesc Med 2011;165:1033–40.

19. Taylor J, Waxman J, Richter S, et al. Evaluation of the effectiveness of anterior cruciate ligament injury prevention programme training components: a systematic review and meta-analysis. Br J Sports Med 2013. [Epub ahead of print]. http://dx.doi.org/10.1136/bjsports-2013-092358.

20. Distefano L, Padua D, Blackburn J, et al. Integrated injury prevention program improves balance and vertical jump height in children. J Strength Cond Res 2010; 24:332–42.

21. Noyes F, Barber-Westin S, Tutalo Smith S, et al. A training program to improve neuromuscular and performance indices in female high school soccer players. J Strength Cond Res 2013;27:340–51.

22. Bartholomew L, Parcel G, Kok G, et al. Planning health promotion programs. 3rd edition. San Francisco: Jossey-Bass; 2011.

23. Klesges L, Estabrooks P, Dzewaltowski D, et al. Beginning with the application in mind: designing and planning health behavior change interventions to enhance dissemination. Ann Behav Med 2005;29:S66–75.

24. Soligard T, Nilstad A, Steffen K, et al. Compliance with a comprehensive warm-up programme to prevent injuries in youth football. Br J Sports Med 2010;44:787–93.

25. Donaldson A, Finch C. Planning for implementation and translation: seek first to understand the end-users' perspectives. Br J Sports Med 2012;46:306–7.

26. Krist M, van Beijsterveldt A, Backx F, et al. Preventive exercises reduced injury-related costs among adult male amateur soccer players: a cluster-randomised trial. J Physiother 2013;59:15–23.

27. Hägglund M, Waldén M, Magnusson H, et al. Injuries affect team performance negatively in professional football: an 11-year follow-up of the UEFA Champions League injury study. Br J Sports Med 2013;47:738–42.

28. Fortington L, Donaldson A, Lathlean T, et al. When "just doing it" is not enough: assessing the fidelity of player performance of an injury prevention exercise program. J Sci Med Sport 2014. [Epub ahead of print].

29. Fixsen DL. Implementation research: a synthesis of the literature. Tampa (FL): Florida Mental Health Institute; 2005. p. 1–125.

ACL Injury and Posttraumatic Osteoarthritis

Steven J. Svoboda, MD

KEYWORDS

- ACL injury • Posttraumatic osteoarthritis • Biomarkers • Biomechanics

KEY POINTS

- Military members are affected by physician-diagnosed osteoarthritis with a higher prevalence than civilian populations.
- Anterior cruciate ligament (ACL) injuries are 10 times more prevalent among military populations than similar civilian cohorts.
- Posttraumatic osteoarthritis (PTOA) occurs in joints after major injuries, such as ACL tears, meniscus tears, or tibial plateau fractures.
- The earliest states of PTOA can be followed and afford the opportunity to study osteoarthritis in a way not possible previously.
- Continuing and future research into the origin of PTOA should focus on natural history studies of young, active patient cohorts who sustain ACL injuries through the earliest stages of the disease (ie, the molecular, preradiographic stage).

OSTEOARTHRITIS BURDEN

Osteoarthritis (OA) is the most common type of arthritis, affecting 27 million people in the United States in 2005.[1] Nearly half of US citizens will develop symptomatic knee OA in the course of their lifetimes with a higher risk in those who are obese or with prior knee joint injury.[2] The rate of physician-diagnosed arthritis is increasing over time and in some populations this is beyond the rate expected due to the aging of the population.[3] It is estimated that 12% of cases of symptomatic OA in the hip, knee, and ankle are due to posttraumatic OA; this is equivalent to 5.6 million cases of posttraumatic osteoarthritis (PTOA) in the United States and a financial burden of more than $3 billion in direct US health care cost for treatment.[4]

Physician-diagnosed OA within the military exists at a much higher incidence than the civilian population.[5] Within the military, musculoskeletal conditions have become

John A. Feagin, Jr. Sports Medicine Fellowship, Keller Army Community Hospital, 900 Washington Road, West Point, NY 10996, USA
E-mail address: steven.j.svoboda.mil@mail.mil

Clin Sports Med 33 (2014) 633–640
http://dx.doi.org/10.1016/j.csm.2014.06.008
0278-5919/14/$ – see front matter © 2014 Elsevier Inc. All rights reserved.

the most common cause of disability leading to medical board evaluation and separation from the service. In particular, back pain and OA were the 2 leading causes of disability for musculoskeletal reasons in 2009.[6] Although devastating injuries such as limb amputations result in greater costs in treatment per patient, there are significantly more injured service members with musculoskeletal injuries not involving amputations such that the cost of their care is the most significant burden to the military health care system. Over a 7-year period, there were over 28,000 anterior cruciate ligament (ACL) injuries in men in the US military and 3500 ACL injuries in women. The rates of the 2 ICD-9 codes for ACL injuries (717.83 and 844.2) were 2.96 and 3.6 cases per 1000 person-years and both represent approximately 10 times greater rates than those reported in similar analyses of representative civilian population data.[7] Clinically, ACL tears are significant causes of knee instability and usually require surgical reconstruction to resolve the knee instability.

PTOA DEFINITION

Traditionally, OA has been defined at the time of radiographic diagnosis using various classification schemes such as Kellgren-Lawrence grade. Posttraumatic OA is a subset of OA that begins with an inciting event such as an intra-articular fracture, a ligament injury, or other cartilage (articular or meniscus) injury within a joint. Earlier-onset symptomatic OA is the outcome depending on the energy and degree of derangement within the joint. PTOA poses a particularly challenging diagnostic conundrum in that defining its incidence and prevalence defies current accepted diagnostic regimens. The definition of OA is a growing challenge within the clinical and research communities. In a clinical setting, this radiographic OA often is associated with symptoms and is defined as symptomatic OA. An alternative definition of OA is self-reported OA, which is based solely on patient report.[8] A recent systematic review confirms the disparity in reporting incident and prevalent OA with pure radiographically diagnosed OA tending to overestimate the disease and that symptomatic OA and self-reported OA have similar incidence and prevalence data in studies.[9]

Distinguishing a joint with primary OA from one with secondary OA is impossible from a plain radiograph taken at one moment in time. Although multiple joint involvement may suggest a primary cause, prior history of joint injury is not always recalled by a patient 20 or 30 years later. Thus, a joint that may have been susceptible to OA due to the patient's OA genotype may develop more severe OA as the result of an inciting injury years before. Currently, other methods for determining OA phenotype are under development. Likely, no one method or classification scheme will serve alone to define the disease; rather, the question being posed will drive the method to use.[8]

ACL INJURY AND PTOA

It is well accepted that the long-term outcome of major knee joint injuries involving the ACL leads to OA. This notion requires further refinement based on evidence provided by longitudinal studies following ACL-injured patients. Neuman and colleagues[10] followed a prospective cohort of ACL-injured patients treated initially without ACL reconstruction for 15 years. At the end of the study period, 94 patients were available for follow-up with 79 having knee injury and osteoarthritis outcome score (KOOS) scores calculated and radiographic examinations performed. Overall, only 16% of radiographed patients had Kellgren-Lawrence grade 2 or greater OA. Those without meniscal tears (n = 44) had no prevalent OA at this follow-up, whereas 37% of patients with meniscus tears either acutely or at later follow-up had radiographic OA. Twenty-three percent of patients did undergo ACL reconstruction at a mean of 4 years after injury because of more than one significant injury, unacceptable activity level, or a reinjury resulting in a symptomatic reparable meniscus tear. ACL-reconstructed patients had a 35% prevalence of tibiofemoral OA, while 46% of patients undergoing ACL reconstruction with a meniscal tear had OA. This study strongly encouraged its participants to give up cutting and pivoting sports and nearly all participated in a neuromuscular rehabilitation program after injury. At enrollment, 92 of 100 subjects played at the highest 2 levels of activity by the International Knee Documentation Committee (IKDC) score, whereas at follow-up, only 56% were participating at such high levels. The original cohort had an average age of 26 years (range, 15–43 years) and 42 years at long-term follow-up, so this does represent a somewhat older cohort. The same cohort was found to have an incidence of patellofemoral (PF) OA of 16% over the study time period with PF OA more frequently having had a meniscal injury and their ACL reconstructed during the time period. PF OA was associated with higher activity level, meniscal injury, flexion and extension deficit, and ACL reconstruction.[11]

The results of this Swedish cohort may be interpreted as a "best case" situation due to several factors. First, subjects were given neuromuscular rehabilitation almost uniformly. Second, all subjects were strongly counseled by their surgeon and treatment staff that they should reduce their activity levels to avoid increased risk of reinjury. Clinically, decision-making with regard to return to play expectations with operative or nonoperative treatment after ACL injury is a shared process with most individuals choosing not to give up high-level cutting and pivoting sports as part of their treatment regimen; thus, it could be expected that most patients will choose surgery. Furthermore, focusing on a young military population with an average age in the early 20s, it seems reasonable that more patients will attempt return to high-level sports versus this Swedish cohort that ranged in age between 15 and 43 years. Thus, it would be logical to expect higher rates of PTOA after ACL injuries in military members.

In a cohort of patients treated with a single bundle ACL reconstruction using a transtibial technique, obesity, increased length of follow-up, grade 2 or greater medial chondrosis, and prior or concurrent medial meniscectomy were found to be most predictive of OA, which occurred in 39% of patients.[12] This cohort was followed a mean of 7.86 years (range, 2.1–20.3 years), which may contribute to underestimating the true prevalence of OA after ACLR.

Whether OA prevalence after ACL injury is related to surgical treatment or to nonoperative management has no clear answer. It is well accepted that reconstruction of the ACL allows return to cutting and pivoting sports and other high-level activities. It is hoped that conferring improved stability on the knee joint will allow for lower incidence of OA after ACL tear, but it may also be that the return to high-level activities on an improved, but not normal, knee increases the forces on the knee that over time lead to OA. Conversely, treating an ACL-injured knee nonoperatively may result in lower OA prevalence owing to a lower activity level; however, if a patient is noncompliant with such an activity prescription, they run the risk of further instability episodes leading to meniscus tears and subsequent degeneration of the articular surface and OA. Which modifiable and nonmodifiable risk factors for OA after ACL tear exist is not completely understood.

Isolated ACL injuries have been studied as a means to eliminate meniscus tears as a confounding variable with regard to OA formation.[13] Patients in a recent study had a diagnostic arthroscopy performed and, based on discussion with the surgeon, were allocated into either a nonoperative group or an ACL-reconstruction using autograft bone-patellar tendon-bone (BTB) either arthroscopically or through a mini-arthrotomy. Although bias was introduced into the study based on the method of allocation, the prevalence of OA in the nonoperative group was 24%, and 45% in the ACL reconstructed group using grade 2 and grade 3 Kellgren-Lawrence rating as the definition of OA. The reason for the high rate of OA may be related to the surgical method in general; the authors pointed to the many changes in ACL technique since this study was conducted between 1989 and 1997. They theorized that as techniques have improved in positioning, fixation, graft choice, and rotational stability, this increased rate of OA seen in this cohort would be decreased in a future study.

Comparison of OA rates after autograft hamstring or BTB ACL reconstructions has shown no difference in radiographic OA at median follow-up of 86 months (25% BTB, 20% Hamstring, P = NS) and this same study supported that OA increased with the presence of meniscal tears.[14] Well-functioning hamstring ACL grafts have been found to have symptomatic OA up to 24% of the time at an average of 10.2 years after ACL reconstruction.[15]

With regard to female sex and high-activity levels (soccer), Lohmander and colleagues[16] found a prevalence of symptomatic knee OA of 42% 12 years after ACL injury in elite-level soccer players. Of these, fully 50% never returned to playing competitive soccer regardless of treatment.

CAUSE OF PTOA AFTER ACL TEAR

Several mechanisms have been implicated in the development of OA after ACL tear: (1) injury to the cartilage directly at the time of ACL rupture, (2) injury to meniscus at the time of ACL tear or later due to chronic instability, (3) increased age at the time of injury, (4) increased shear forces and supraphysiologic compressive forces on discrete regions of the joint surface, and (5) inflammatory changes caused by the acute hemarthrosis. Although abnormal mechanical forces can directly cause joint damage, it is likely that they also contribute to a cascade of biochemical events due to mechanosensitive inflammatory and repair signals.[17] A critical concept is that OA is not simply a disease of cartilage. OA should be considered in the context of the whole joint as a single functional organ, including cartilage, bone, synovium, and ligaments. Thus, although it is conceptually easy to see mechanical forces leading to changes in chondrocytes within cartilage as one example, synoviocytes within the synovium of articular joints also may play a role in the development of PTOA.

PARADIGM SHIFT IN THE STUDY OF OA

With the acceleration of understanding of joint biology presaged by molecular biological techniques developed in the disciplines of proteomics and genomics, a paradigm shift is occurring in the study of OA. Wherein phenotypic groups of OA have been previously categorized by radiographic findings, current opinion is that radiographic changes associated with all forms of OA are the last to occur in the chain of events arising from the initiation of disease. At the point that osteophytes, joint space narrowing, subchondral sclerosis, and flattening of joint surfaces occur, the joint is at its end stage. PTOA treatment in its end state is no different than any other form of OA—total joint arthroplasty. The novel concept with PTOA lies in its earliest state, a period when the disease is silent with regard to symptoms, yet the manifestations of OA begin at this initial time point. Thus, for a pilon fracture or tibial plateau fracture, one modifiable risk factor would be how well the articular surface is reconstituted. For a major ligament injury, the earliest modifiable risk factor (besides prevention) may be joint aspiration to remove a hemarthrosis or an injection of an as-yet undefined agent that may be able to minimize the acute changes in the joint that lead to chondrocyte functional changes.

Although PTOA may represent a small proportion of all OA disease, it is proving to be the focus of defining the earliest etiologic changes that occur in a joint at risk for OA. Major joint injury is typically a well-defined event that uniformly brings the injured patients to the attention of the health care system. This event affords an opportunity to both study the earliest point in the disease process and potentially allow early treatments for PTOA to be provided as more is learned of the early disease. It has been suggested that PTOA be considered the same as cardiovascular disease, where early disease can be measured through surrogates, such as blood pressure and serum cholesterol levels.[18] Thus, the radiographic stage of the PTOA would be akin to symptomatic ischemic disease, like a myocardial infarction, with these representing the end stage of these disease processes. The preradiographic stage of PTOA (ie, when it can be observed through surrogates such as bone scan, magnetic resonance imaging [MRI]) is similar to when cardiovascular disease can be defined by cardiac catheterization or blood pressure measurement. Finally, the earliest stage of these 2 diseases would be defined as a molecular stage, where it may be diagnosed at its earliest stages. This molecular stage would afford the opportunity to intervene in the disease process when potentially reversible disease states can be modified by external inputs.

KNOWLEDGE GAPS IN PTOA
Early Diagnosis Knowledge Gaps

Radiographs
As the aforementioned discussion of the late clinical outcome of PTOA after ACL tear centered on radiographic characteristics of the disease, the shortcomings of using radiographs as a disease endpoint should be pointed out. First, radiographic evaluation of OA has commonly centered on clinical diagnostic criteria, such as Kellgren-Lawrence or Outerbridge classification schemes. These systems are relatively insensitive to early changes in OA and tend to break subjects down into one of only several categories. In addition to this insensitivity to the progressive nature of the disease, there is also interobserver disagreement in classifying individual cases.

Standardized, weight-bearing radiographs registered from one time point to the next are critical for accurate analysis of disease progression. Given the relative lack of standardized technique required to accurately measure joint space width (JSW) in the clinical state, classification schemes such as Kellgren-Lawrence may be the only feasible classification method. As the National Institutes of Health (NIH)-sponsored Osteoarthritis Initiative has done, standardizing technique across multiple centers using positioning equipment such as a Synaflexer Frame (Synarc, Inc, San Francisco, CA, USA) would allow comparisons to be made more accurately across more and larger cohorts and, most importantly, allow the accurate measurement of JSW over serial radiographs.[19]

Advanced imaging
Although the use of such standardized radiographs allows the earliest measurement of JSW changes, JSW is primarily a measurement in the change in articular cartilage thickness in early OA. Radiographs poorly provide information on the synovium, meniscus, ligaments, and even articular cartilage. MRI provides the ability to image all of these structures and, with specific sequences, may even provide detail on the actual functioning of that tissue. For example, the bone bruise noted on the lateral femoral condyle and the posterior border of the lateral tibial plateau is a pathognomonic sign of an ACL tear. Further work is being performed that attempts to quantify the volume of a bone bruise and, thus, provide a gauge of the degree of injury imparted

to the bone. Should reproducible methods become available to quantify these bone bruises, it may be possible to use this as a tool in predicting the expected speed and degree of PTOA development that may occur after an injury.

Surrogate markers

Markers of physiologic processes that vary in conjunction with a specific disease state can be described as biomarkers. Radiographs and MRIs can be considered a specific type—imaging biomarkers. Other biomarkers are typically obtained from the body directly as biospecimens, such as blood and serum, synovial fluid, and other tissue samples. With appropriate validation through research, biomarkers may be found that act as surrogates for the progression of a disease process. Thus, coronary artery disease risk can be calculated via surrogates, such as blood pressure, serum cholesterol, and risk factors like smoking. Actual coronary angiography, the gold standard for diagnosis of coronary artery disease, is not necessary when assessing risk of this disease. Similarly, although radiographs are known to be surrogates for OA, as discussed earlier, they are insensitive to early disease states. MRI affords the opportunity for earlier diagnosis of the OA phenotype, but MRI scans are expensive, and appropriate imaging capability is not available everywhere.

A gap exists in the knowledge base that allows clinicians to follow the early stages of OA. Furthermore, a gap exists in the treatments available for joints in the earliest stages of OA. The OA Biomarkers Initiative was instituted by the OA Biomarkers Network and the Osteoarthritis Research Society International and consisted of educational and goal-setting symposia. Significant emphasis was placed on biomarker validation as part of this ongoing effort. Notably, the BIPED classification criteria were created that define biomarkers into 5 categories: *b*urden of disease, *i*nvestigative, *p*rognostic, *e*fficacy of intervention, and *d*iagnostic markers.[20] The framework of the BIPED classification allows for the creation of well-designed, iterative research to answer the major questions in early OA development. With support of the NIH, the Osteoarthritis Initiative was created and serves as a repository of prospectively collected data in subjects with OA, including biospecimens, imaging both radiographs and 3-T MRI, and clinical data.

Recent work with West Point cadets has shed light on the changes of serum biomarkers of cartilage turnover that occur after ACL injury.[21] Serum was collected on entry to the United States Military Academy and again just before graduation 4 years later. The serum from cadets sustaining ACL injuries during their time at West Point was compared with a group of matched control cadets not sustaining significant joint injury during their 4 years at West Point. Controls were matched to cases by age, sex, and body mass index. Markers associated with synthesis of type II collagen (CPII) and aggrecan (CS846) as well as markers associated with degradation of type I and type II collagen (C1,2C, and C2C) were measured at the 2 time points. Significant differences in C1,2C ($P = .042$), C2C ($P = .006$), and CS846 ($P = .002$) were found over time in the ACL-injured group compared with the uninjured control group. Ratios of markers of degradation to synthesis were also analyzed. The change in the ratio of C2C:CPII was found to be significantly different between injured and noninjured subjects ($P = .013$) but not in the ratio of C1,2C:CPII. Comparison of the preinjury ratios between groups found no significant differences, whereas the postinjury ratios were significantly different for both ratios. This statistically significant difference between the change in the ratio of C2C:CPII in the 2 groups suggests an uncoupling of synthesis and degradation of common cartilage constituents. Future study of longer-term changes in these serum biomarkers are necessary to see if this trend continues over time. Commercially available ELISA kits available today for cartilage research cannot have their results compared across different lots owing predominantly to the fact that they have not been applied against large cohorts of subjects so that results from kits from different lots have not been normalized. A potential strength of analyzing ratios lies in the fact that they are unitless and eliminate the need to use biomarker kits obtained from the same production lot—a practical difficulty of biomarker research in its current state.

Treatment Knowledge Gaps

For further advancement of treatment interventions, some modification to treatment outcomes must be made. Current requirements by the Food and Drug Administration call for new treatments of OA to show radiographic improvement to be called efficacious. This call for new treatments has had the effect of driving the pharmaceutical industry from the field because many treatment paradigms will call for interventions before any evidence of classic OA. Proposed treatments have ranged anywhere from simple joint aspiration at the time of injury to the injection of novel compounds that intervene in the inflammatory cascade, such as IL-1RA and other targets. As the initial injury state may be found to be a primary cause of the eventual PTOA, it may be that more urgent intervention at the time of injury becomes the new paradigm as more is learned about the earliest stages of PTOA.

SUMMARY

Continued development and validation of quantitative imaging and biochemical assessment techniques are critical research priorities to lead to improved diagnosis and treatment of PTOA. There is also a compelling need to advance understanding of how mechanical joint injuries lead to joint degeneration, and to define the roles of acute joint damage and post–joint injury incongruity and instability as etiologic factors leading to development of OA.[22] As OA occurs more frequently in the military population and ACL tears are endemic to the military, it is essential that the military become more active in funding research and seeking novel research cohorts to help solve some of the most fundamental problems in PTOA. The military population, while deeply affected by PTOA, may also prove to be pivotal in determining improved diagnostic techniques and treatment interventions to help minimize the long-term effects of this disease.

REFERENCES

1. Lawrence RC, Felson DT, Helmick CG, et al. Estimates of the prevalence of arthritis and other rheumatic conditions in the United States. Part II. Arthritis Rheum 2008; 58(1):26–35.
2. Murphy L, Schwartz TA, Helmick CG, et al. Lifetime risk of symptomatic knee osteoarthritis. Arthritis Rheum 2008;59(9):1207–13.
3. Kopec JA, Rahman MM, Sayre EC, et al. Trends in physician-diagnosed osteoarthritis incidence in an administrative database in British Columbia, Canada, 1996-1997 through 2003-2004. Arthritis Rheum 2008;59(7):929–34.
4. Brown TD, Johnston RC, Saltzman CL, et al. Posttraumatic osteoarthritis: a first estimate of incidence, prevalence, and burden of disease. J Orthop Trauma 2006; 20(10):739–44.
5. Cameron KL, Hsiao MS, Owens BD, et al. Incidence of physician-diagnosed osteoarthritis among active duty United States military service members. Arthritis Rheum 2011;63(10):2974–82.

6. Patzkowski JC, Rivera JC, Ficke JR, et al. The changing face of disability in the US Army: the Operation Enduring Freedom and Operation Iraqi Freedom effect. J Am Acad Orthop Surg 2012;20(Suppl 1):S23–30.

7. Owens BD, Mountcastle SB, Dunn WR, et al. Incidence of anterior cruciate ligament injury among active duty U.S. military servicemen and servicewomen. Mil Med 2007;172(1):90–1.

8. Nelson AE, Jordan JM. Defining osteoarthritis: a moving target. Osteoarthritis Cartilage 2012;20(1):1–3.

9. Pereira D, Peleteiro B, Araujo J, et al. The effect of osteoarthritis definition on prevalence and incidence estimates: a systematic review. Osteoarthritis Cartilage 2011;19(11):1270–85.

10. Neuman P, Englund M, Kostogiannis I, et al. Prevalence of tibiofemoral osteoarthritis 15 years after nonoperative treatment of anterior cruciate ligament injury: a prospective cohort study. Am J Sports Med 2008;36(9):1717–25.

11. Neuman P, Kostogiannis I, Friden T, et al. Patellofemoral osteoarthritis 15 years after anterior cruciate ligament injury–a prospective cohort study. Osteoarthritis Cartilage 2009;17(3):284–90.

12. Li RT, Lorenz S, Xu Y, et al. Predictors of radiographic knee osteoarthritis after anterior cruciate ligament reconstruction. Am J Sports Med 2011;39(12):2595–603.

13. Kessler MA, Behrend H, Henz S, et al. Function, osteoarthritis and activity after ACL-rupture: 11 years follow-up results of conservative versus reconstructive treatment. Knee Surg Sports Traumatol Arthrosc 2008;16(5):442–8.

14. Liden M, Sernert N, Rostgard-Christensen L, et al. Osteoarthritic changes after anterior cruciate ligament reconstruction using bone-patellar tendon-bone or hamstring tendon autografts: a retrospective, 7-year radiographic and clinical follow-up study. Arthroscopy 2008;24(8):899–908.

15. Struewer J, Ziring E, Frangen TM, et al. Clinical outcome and prevalence of osteoarthritis after isolated anterior cruciate ligament reconstruction using hamstring graft: follow-up after two and ten years. Int Orthop 2013;37(2):271–7.

16. Lohmander LS, Ostenberg A, Englund M, et al. High prevalence of knee osteoarthritis, pain, and functional limitations in female soccer players twelve years after anterior cruciate ligament injury. Arthritis Rheum 2004;50(10):3145–52.

17. Olson SA, Horne P, Furman B, et al. The role of cytokines in posttraumatic arthritis. J Am Acad Orthop Surg 2014;22(1):29–37.

18. Kraus VB, Nevitt M, Sandell LJ. Summary of the OA biomarkers workshop 2009–biochemical biomarkers: biology, validation, and clinical studies. Osteoarthritis Cartilage 2010;18(6):742–5.

19. Charles HC, Kraus VB, Ainslie M, et al. Optimization of the fixed-flexion knee radiograph. Osteoarthritis Cartilage 2007;15(11):1221–4.

20. Bauer DC, Hunter DJ, Abramson SB, et al. Classification of osteoarthritis biomarkers: a proposed approach. Osteoarthritis Cartilage 2006;14(8):723–7.

21. Svoboda SJ, Harvey TM, Owens BD, et al. Changes in serum biomarkers of cartilage turnover after anterior cruciate ligament injury. Am J Sports Med 2013;41(9):2108–16.

22. Chu CR, Beynnon BD, Buckwalter JA, et al. Closing the gap between bench and bedside research for early arthritis therapies (EARTH): report from the AOSSM/NIH U-13 Post-Joint Injury Osteoarthritis Conference II. Am J Sports Med 2011;39(7):1569–78.

Meniscal Repair and Transplantation in the Military Active-duty Population

CrossMark

John-Paul Rue, MD[a,b,*], Adam Pickett, MD[c]

KEYWORDS

- Knee • Meniscal repair • Arthroscopy • Military

KEY POINTS

- Meniscal tears are described by their location and morphology.
- The location of the tear in relation to the vascular supply is the most important intrinsic factor in healing.
- Augmentation techniques are performed to enhance the local healing environment by introducing factors found in the peripheral blood, such as growth factors, fibrin, and platelets, to the site of repair.
- General anesthesia or regional anesthesia may be used when indicated.
- Meniscal transplantation has an undetermined role in the active-duty population and has been traditionally been considered a "salvage" procedure.

INTRODUCTION

Injuries to the menisci that necessitate surgery are commonly reported in both the general and physically active populations. In active-duty US military service members, the incidence of meniscal tears is reported to be 10 times higher than that of the civilian population. Male gender, increasing age, and service in the Army or the Marine Corps are factors associated with a higher incidence of meniscal tears within the military.[1]

In the past meniscal tears were treated with a complete meniscectomy until Fairbank[2] noticed in 1948 that, over time, postmeniscectomy knees showed joint space

Funding Sources: None.
Conflict of Interest: None.
[a] Uniformed Services University of the Health Services, Bethesda, MD, USA; [b] Department of Orthopaedics and Sports Medicine, Naval Health Clinic Annapolis, US Naval Academy, 250 Wood Road, Annapolis, MD 21402-5050, USA; [c] Department of Orthopaedics, Walter Reed National Military Medical Center, 8901 Wisconsin Avenue, Bethesda, MD 20814, USA
* Corresponding author. Department of Orthopaedics and Sports Medicine, Naval Health Clinic Annapolis, US Naval Academy, 250 Wood Road, Annapolis, MD 21402-5050.
E-mail address: john-paul.rue@med.navy.mil

narrowing, femoral flattening, and osteophyte formation. Since that time the morbidities associated with complete meniscectomy have been well documented: mainly the development of knee osteoarthritis. Thus attention has been turned to meniscus preservation and recent technological advances have made meniscal repairs easier and stronger.

ANATOMY AND BIOMECHANICS

The knee menisci are a pair of wedge-shaped semilunar cartilages that are interposed between the femoral condyles and tibial plateau.[3] The medial meniscus is approximately 4 to 5 cm in length, oval, connected to deep medial collateral ligament (MCL), and serves as a secondary stabilizer in the knee. The lateral meniscus is approximately 3 to 4 cm in length, circular, and not connected to the joint capsule within the popliteal hiatus, allowing 11 mm motion compared with 5 mm of motion in the medial meniscus.[4] Their blood supply originates from a perimeniscal capillary plexus originating in the capsular and synovial tissues of the joint supplies the peripheral 10% to 25% arising from the medial and lateral geniculate arteries.[5]

The menisci are composed of mostly type I collagen fibers arranged in a circumferential pattern[6] that transform axial load into hoop stresses.[7–9] There is a linear correlation between the increase in peak pressure on the joint surfaces and the percentage of fibers disrupted.[10] Removal of the meniscus completely reduces joint contact area by 75% and increases peak load stresses on the articular cartilage by 235%.[11] The menisci also play roles in shock absorption,[12] joint stabilization,[4] joint lubrication,[13] articular cartilage nutrition,[14] and proprioception.[15]

MENISCAL TEARS

Meniscal tears are described by their location and morphology. Each meniscus is divided into 12 zones, called Cooper zones, according to their location.[16] The 4 longitudinal zones are divided based on their proximity to the vascularity of meniscus (eg, red-red, red-white, or white-white). The 3 radial zones divide each meniscus into anterior/posterior meniscal horns and meniscal body. Tears are also described by their morphology, and types include horizontal; bucket handle; longitudinal (ie, vertical); oblique (ie, flap); radial; and complex, which consists of a combination of different tear morphologies.

REPAIR INDICATIONS

The location of the tear in relation to the vascular supply is the most important intrinsic factor in healing (**Table 1**). Meniscal repairs for tears in the red-red or red-white zone, Cooper zones 0 to 2, or that have a meniscal rim width of less than 4 mm, have the highest success rates.[17,18] As patients age, the meniscal tissue has less cellularity and a decreased healing response than tissue from younger patients[24] and studies have shown that younger patients have higher rates of successful repairs for tears that extend into the avascular zone of the meniscus.[19–21] In the young active-duty population, a repair should be attempted because the chance of healing outweighs the potential risks of the procedure and the long-term sequelae of meniscectomy early in life.[20]

Tear morphology is another factor determining a successful meniscal repair. Longitudinal and bucket handle tears are commonly repaired because they are amenable to suture fixation. Radial tears have identical tibiofemoral contact mechanics to a complete meniscectomy that may return to normal once the tear is repaired.[25,26] Partial

Table 1
Significant and insignificant factors affecting healing rates of meniscal repairs in the literature

Author, Year	Type of Study	Significant Factors (P Value)	Insignificant Factors (P Value)
Scott et al,[17] 1986	Prospective cohort of 178 meniscal repairs in 167 patients	Tear within 2 mm of peripheral rim ($P = .03$); Concomitant ligament (ACL or PCL) reconstruction ($P = .0001$)	Perimeniscal synovial membrane dissection ($P = .06$); Single vs double longitudinal tears ($P = .07$); Length of tear >20 mm ($P = .09$); Lateral vs medial meniscus ($P = .10$); Age of patient >35 y ($P = .27$); Time from injury to surgery >3 wk ($P = .44$); Distance of tear from the posterior horn ($P = .47$); Tears >8 wk from injury ($P<.25$)
Cannon & Vittori,[18] 1992	Case-control study of 68 meniscus repairs with a concomitant ligament reconstruction vs 22 meniscus repairs in ligamentously stable knees	Concomitant ligament reconstruction ($P = .00005$); Lateral vs medial meniscus ($P<.04$); Tear within 4 mm of meniscal rim; Tear length <4 cm	—
Noyes & Barber-Westin,[19] 2002	Retrospective review of 71 meniscal repairs in patients <20 y old	Age of patient <20 y; Concomitant ligament reconstruction	—
Rubman et al,[20] 1998	Retrospective review of 180 meniscal repairs located in the avascular zone of the meniscus	Lateral vs medial meniscus ($P = .008$); Time from repair to follow-up arthroscopy >12 mo ($P = .02$)	Time from injury to meniscal repair ($P = .06$); Age of patient >25 y
Tengrootenhuysen et al,[21] 2011	Retrospective review of 119 meniscal repairs	Concomitant ligament reconstruction ($P = .046$); Time from injury to surgery <6 wk ($P = .001$); Age of patient ($P = .024$)	Age of patient >25 y; Tear location, zone 0 vs zone 1; Medial vs lateral meniscus
Kimura et al,[22] 1995	Retrospective cohort of 46 out of 137 consecutive meniscal repairs	Concomitant ligament reconstruction ($P<.005$)	Length of tear; Pedicle synovial transplant
Gallacher et al,[23] 2012	Case-control study of 24 patients who had meniscus repair before ACL reconstruction vs 148 patients who had concomitant ACL reconstruction with meniscus repair	Concomitant ACL reconstruction ($P = .05$)	—

Abbreviations: ACL, anterior cruciate ligament; PCL, posterior cruciate ligament.

radial tears, located in the avascular zone; are typically debrided, whereas complete tears may be repaired or stabilized, especially in a young patient.[25,26] Degenerative or complex tears tend to be associated with chronic damage to the meniscus and are typically debrided.[18] Horizontal tears are typically not repaired because they are frequently degenerative and the tear morphology is not amenable to stable suture constructs or healing (**Fig. 1**).[17,19]

Anterior cruciate ligament (ACL) tear is the most common injury that occurs concurrently with meniscal tear. Tears of the lateral meniscus are generally found following acute ACL rupture, likely resulting from the initial injury, and have a simple morphology. In contrast, tears of the medial meniscus are often found in chronically ACL-deficient knees, likely resulting from the increased instability, and are typically degenerative and complex. Meniscal repairs performed concomitantly with ACL reconstruction have been shown to be as successful[27] or significantly more successful than meniscal repair alone,[17,18,21,23] which may be the result of the release of blood and other healing factors into the joint during the ACL reconstruction.

The influence of the tear length on the failure rate is not clear. Some investigators have found that failures occurred significantly earlier in tears larger than 4 cm,[18,28] whereas others could not prove an association between the failure rate and the length of the tear.[22] Timing of repair is also controversial. Some studies report increased rates when repaired within 6 weeks of injury,[21] whereas others have shown no difference of timing on healing rates.[17–20,27]

REPAIR TECHNIQUES

At present, there are 3 repair techniques commonly described: inside out, outside in, and all inside (**Table 2**). Regardless of the technique used, the orientation of the suture across the meniscus has an effect on the strength of the repair. Mechanical studies have shown that vertical mattress sutures provide stronger fixation than horizontal mattress sutures.[38–40] The vertical mattress sutures capture the more abundant and robust circumferential fibers of the meniscus, whereas the horizontal mattress sutures align in parallel and can be pulled out (**Figs. 2** and **3**).

The inside-out technique has long been considered to be the gold standard for meniscal repair. With the inside-out technique, sutures are inserted into the meniscus using a needle cannula under arthroscopic visualization. There are specific cannulas based on the location of the tear (zone specific) that bend the needle to engage the

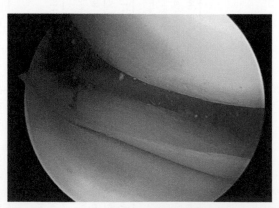

Fig. 1. A meniscus tear that is a good candidate for repair because it is located in the red-white zone, is nondegenerative, and longitudinal in morphology.

Table 2
Success rates of various meniscal repair techniques

Author, Year	Type of Study	Techniques Evaluated	Mean Follow-up	Success Rate (%)	Mean Subjective Scores (If Reported)	Complication Rate (Most Common Complication)
Grant et al,[29] 2012	Systematic review of 19 studies using inside-out or all-inside technique for isolated meniscus repairs	Inside out All inside	— —	83 81	Lysholm, 87.8; Tegner, 5.6 Lysholm, 90.2; Tegner, 5.5	9% (nerve irritation/injury) 2% (nerve irritation/injury)
Abdelkafy et al,[30] 2007	Retrospective review of 41 meniscal repairs performed with outside-in technique	Outside in	11.71 y	88	Lysholm, 87.29; SF-36, 85.73	No complications reported
Barrett et al,[31] 1997	Prospective cohort of 24 meniscal repairs with concurrent ACL reconstruction	Second generation, all inside	17 mo	81	Lysholm, 87.29; SF-36, 85.37	4% (infection)
Escalas et al,[32] 1997	Prospective cohort of 20 meniscal repairs	Second generation, all inside	12 mo	95	—	No complications reported
Gill & Diduch,[33] 2002	Retrospective review of 32 meniscal tears with concurrent ACL reconstruction	Third generation, all inside	2.3 y	91	—	No complications reported
Lee & Diduch,[34] 2005	Extended follow-up review of the 32 patients surveyed in the previous study	Third generation, all inside	6.6 y	71	—	No complications reported
Gifstad et al,[35] 2007	Retrospective review of 118 meniscal repairs	Third generation, all inside	4.7 y	59	Lysholm, 85	3% (displacement of arrows)
Haas et al,[36] 2005	Prospective cohort of 42 meniscal repairs	Fourth generation, all inside	24.3 mo	87	Lysholm 93.73	—
Quinby et al,[37] 2006	Retrospective review of 54 meniscal tears with concurrent ACL reconstruction	Fourth generation, all inside	34.8 mo	90.7	—	—

Abbreviation: SF-36, Short Form 36.

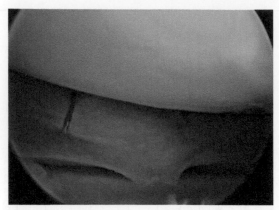

Fig. 2. A meniscus tear repaired with vertical mattress sutures.

tear based on its location in the meniscus (**Fig. 4**). Once the needle has been introduced, an incision is made down onto the capsule through the appropriate interval, generally one-third above and two-thirds below the joint line to accommodate the trajectory of the sutures being passed. The medial interval is between the MCL and the medial head of the gastrocnemius, retracting the pes posteriorly and protecting the saphenous nerve. The dissection should split the iliotibial band laterally and continue between the lateral collateral ligament and the lateral head of the gastrocnemius. A sterile spoon, meniscal repair retractor, or a vaginal speculum may assist in retrieving the needles and protect the posterior neurovascular structures. Make sure to tie sutures onto the capsule with the knee in relative extension to prevent capture of the posterior capsule of the knee as it folds in flexion, thus limiting extension.[41] Last, close the skin incision over the tied sutures.

The outside-in technique is an effective alternative to the inside-out technique, particularly for anterior horn meniscal tears. To perform the outside-in technique, first pass a spinal needle from outside the knee across the tear. Keep the spinal needle anterior to the gastrocnemius to avoid piercing the neurovascular structures. Next, thread a 0 PDS suture through the spinal needle and pull it through the anterior medial portal with a grasper. Repeat the first two steps adjacent to the first entry point to create a suture bridge across the repair site. The 2 PDS sutures are then tied together

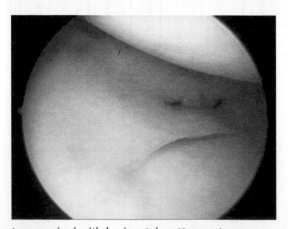

Fig. 3. A meniscus tear repaired with horizontal mattress sutures.

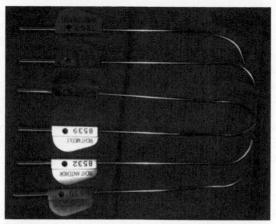

Fig. 4. The zone-specific cannulas used for the inside-out meniscus repair technique.

or may be exchanged for a nonabsorbable suture. Dissection is then made to the capsule over the suture, which is tied together over the capsule (**Fig. 5**).[42]

Both of these techniques have proved to be effective, with 12% to 17% failure rates.[29,30] However, complications to the neurovascular structures surrounding the knee are documented with both of these techniques.[42,43] The popliteal artery is at risk posteriorly with hematoma, aneurysm, and pseudoaneurysm described in the literature.[44] The common peroneal nerve[45] and the lateral geniculate artery[46] are at risk laterally. The saphenous nerve is at risk medially with either neuroma formation or irritation described in the literature.

All-inside techniques were developed to mitigate these complications. First-generation all-inside devices[47] involved the insertion of curved suture hooks through accessory posterior portals to pass sutures across the tear. The technique was technically demanding and continued to place the neurovascular structures at risk so second-generation devices were developed, which were the first to have technique-specific devices placed across the tear and anchored peripherally. Each anchor had 1 suture, and 2 adjacent sutures would be tied together arthroscopically.

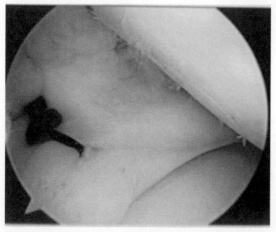

Fig. 5. A meniscal tear in the anterior body of the meniscus repaired with an outside-in technique.

Third-generation all-inside repair devices were developed to create more compression across the repair. They involve the insertion of rigid arrow or screw implants made of absorbable polymers into the peripheral soft tissues. Even though initial success rates were promising,[33] on long-term follow-up success rates significantly declined.[34] These devises were also prone to break,[48] migrate, and damage articular cartilage.[49]

The fourth-generation and current-generation devices were designed to be flexible, low profile, and suture based to allow for compression and variable tension across the meniscal tear. These devices have biomechanical characteristics that are comparable with inside-out techniques and significantly better than previous generation all-inside constructs.[50,51] Early clinical results are showing a comparable overall success rate with inside-out suture repairs.[36,37]

ENHANCEMENT

Augmentation techniques are performed to enhance the local healing environment by introducing factors found in the peripheral blood, such as growth factors, fibrin, and platelets, to the site of repair. One method is to use a meniscal rasp or arthroscopic shaver to abrade the meniscal-synovial junction and induce bleeding near the site of repair. Meniscal abrasion has been shown to promote the healing response through the expression of cytokines (**Fig. 6**).[52]

Exogenous fibrin clots may be useful in the setting of isolated meniscal repair. They are created by spinning autologous blood in a glass tube until a clot is formed, which is then placed at the repair site.[53] This technique has shown good results; however, it is technically challenging with limited application in practice.

REHABILITATION

The postoperative limitations of meniscal repair are markedly greater than those of partial meniscectomy, and rehabilitation generally follows standard principles. For the first 4 to 6 weeks the patient can be either weight bearing as tolerated (WBAT) or protected weight bearing and should avoid deep flexion[54–56] and internal and external rotation of the tibia in order to avoid stress on the repair.[56] After this initial period, a formal physical therapy program is initiated focused on protecting the integrity of the repair, avoiding disuse changes in bone and soft tissue, and restoring and

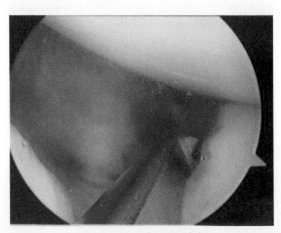

Fig. 6. The surgeon preparing the meniscal surfaces and the meniscal-synovial junction with a rasp.

preserving knee range of motion and strength. At 4 months the patient may begin running, cutting, deep squats, or knee flexion.

However, recent research has shown no difference in failure rates comparing conservative rehabilitation protocols with accelerated rehabilitation protocols[57,58] in which patients were allowed immediate, full weight bearing after surgery and return to sports when tolerated. When patients have concurrent ACL reconstruction, they should follow standard ACL rehabilitation protocols.[59]

AUTHORS' PREFERRED TECHNIQUE

General anesthesia or regional anesthesia may be used when indicated. Patients are placed in the supine position with either the foot of the bed lowered or not. Either positioning technique is acceptable as long as it allows access to the medial and lateral side of the knee. At the surgeons' discretion, a well-padded tourniquet may be used on the operative thigh placed proximal enough to avoid draping out the surgical field. The operative leg is placed in either a leg holder or a lateral leg post, which allows sufficient flexion and access to both the medial and lateral aspects of the knee. We prefer to position the patient with the foot of the bed lowered and the operative extremity placed in a leg holder with a tourniquet on the proximal thigh. Standard prepping and draping is then performed with care taken to ensure that there is adequate visualization and access to both the medial and lateral aspects of the knee.

After diagnostic arthroscopy, the tear is evaluated to determine whether repair is indicated. Our repair indications are peripheral tears with a maximum rim width of 4 mm with sufficient viable tissue to hold a repair securely. Indications are expanded when meniscal repairs are performed concomitantly with an ACL, or for younger patients. If repair is indicated, the meniscal surfaces are prepared with gentle and minimal debridement using a motorized shaver device and the surrounding meniscal-synovial junction is rasped. The repair is performed with a fourth-generation all-inside system using vertical mattress suture techniques. The surgeon should direct the suture repair devices in a direction that is generally away from the neurovascular structures and appropriate fat-pad debridement at the portal sites assists the surgeon in introducing the device into the knee and improves visualization. As an alternative, combinations of vertical mattress, horizontal mattress, or oblique suture repair patterns may be required based on the tear pattern, location, and visibility to ensure a stable repair. The portal sites are closed and the knee is bandaged with fluffs, web

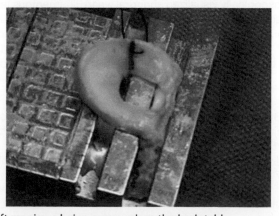

Fig. 7. An allograft meniscus being prepared on the back table.

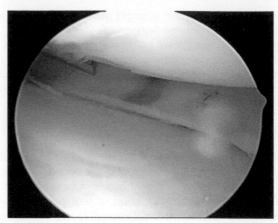

Fig. 8. An allograft meniscus transplant secured to the joint capsule with multiple vertical mattress sutures.

roll, and a loosely wrapped ace wrap, followed by a compression stocking and cryotherapy.

After surgery, a standard rehabilitation protocol is followed. Immediately the operative extremity is WBAT in extension, flexion is restricted to less than 90° with no weight bearing in flexion for 6 to 8 weeks. After these initial restrictions patients may begin to increase their activity levels, but hamstring slides and wall squats are avoided for 2 to 3 months.

MENISCAL TRANSPLANTATION

Meniscal transplantation has an undetermined role in the active-duty population and has been traditionally been considered a salvage procedure (**Figs. 7** and **8**). The surgeon should have an extensive discussion with the service member before considering the procedure about reasonable expectations for outcomes and the future implications for continued military service. It is indicated in an active, young patient (less than 50 years of age) who has undergone either a complete or near-complete meniscectomy with pain in the involved compartment without moderate to severe arthrosis (less than 2 to 3 mm of radiographic joint space narrowing or Outerbridge grade I or II arthroscopically visualized chondral wear), ligamentous laxity, or malalignment.[60] The patient should also discontinue physical activity for 6 to 9 months to allow the meniscus to incorporate and may have to limit lifetime physical activity to light activity. Results of meniscal transplantation vary from 100%[61] to 12.5%[62] with an average of more than 60% of patients having pain-free knees with daily living.

REFERENCES

1. Jones JC, Burks R, Owens BD, et al. Incidence and risk factors associated with meniscal injuries among active-duty US military service members. J Athl Train 2012;47(1):67–73.
2. Fairbank TJ. Knee joint changes after meniscectomy. J Bone Joint Surg Br 1948; 30(4):664–70.
3. Messner K, Gao J. The menisci of the knee joint. Anatomical and functional characteristics, and a rationale for clinical treatment. J Anat 1998;193(Pt 2): 161–78.

4. Shoemaker SC, Markolf KL. The role of the meniscus in the anterior-posterior stability of the loaded anterior cruciate deficient knee. J Bone Joint Surg Am 1986;68(1):71–9.
5. Arnoczky SP, Warren RF. Microvasculature of the human meniscus. Am J Sports Med 1982;10(2):90–5.
6. McDevitt C, Webber RJ. The ultrastructure and biochemistry of meniscal cartilage. Clin Orthop Relat Res 1990;252:8–18.
7. Ahmed AM, Burke DL. In-vitro measurement of static pressure distribution in synovial joints: part I. Tibial surface of the knee. J Biomech Eng 1983;105(3):216–25.
8. Thompson WO, Thaete FL, Fu FH, et al. Tibial meniscal dynamics using three-dimensional reconstruction of magnetic resonance images. Am J Sports Med 1991;19:210–6.
9. Krause WR, Pope MH, Johnson RJ, et al. Mechanical changes in the knee after meniscectomy. J Bone Joint Surg Am 1976;58A:599–603.
10. Bedi A, Kelly NH, Baad M, et al. Dynamic contact mechanics of the medial meniscus as a function of radial tear, repair, and partial meniscectomy. J Bone Joint Surg Am 2010;92(6):1398–408.
11. Baratz ME, Fu FH, Mengato R. Meniscal tears: the effect of meniscectomy and of repair on intraarticular contact areas and stress in the human knee. Am J Sports Med 1986;14:270–4.
12. Voloshin AS, Wosk J. Shock absorption of meniscectomized and painful knees: a comparative in vivo study. J Biomed Eng 1983;5(2):157–61.
13. MacConaill MA. The movements of bones and joints; the synovial fluid and its assistants. J Bone Joint Surg Br 1950;32B(2):244–52.
14. Renström P, Johnson RJ. Anatomy and biomechanics of the menisci. Clin Sports Med 1990;9(3):523–38.
15. Zimny ML, Albright DJ, Dabezies E. Mechanoreceptors in the human medial meniscus. Acta Anat (Basel) 1988;133(1):35–40.
16. Cooper DE, Arnoczky SP, Warren RF. Meniscal repair. Clin Sports Med 1991;10(3):529–48.
17. Scott GA, Jolly BL, Henning CE. Combined posterior incision and arthroscopic intra-articular repair of the meniscus: an examination of factors affecting healing. J Bone Joint Surg Am 1986;68(6):847–61.
18. Cannon WD Jr, Vittori JM. The incidence of healing in arthroscopic meniscal repairs in anterior cruciate ligament-reconstructed knees versus stable knees. Am J Sports Med 1992;20(2):176–81.
19. Noyes FR, Barber-Westin SD. Arthroscopic repair of meniscal tears extending into the avascular zone in patients younger than twenty years of age. Am J Sports Med 2002;30(4):589–600.
20. Rubman MH, Noyes FR, Barber-Westin SD. Arthroscopic repair of meniscal tears that extend into the avascular zone: a review of 198 single and complex tears. Am J Sports Med 1998;26(1):87–95.
21. Tengrootenhuysen M, Meermans G, Pittoors K, et al. Long-term outcome after meniscal repair. Knee Surg Sports Traumatol Arthrosc 2011;19(2):236–41.
22. Kimura M, Shirakura K, Hasegawa A, et al. Second look arthroscopy after meniscal repair. Factors affecting the healing rate. Clin Orthop Relat Res 1995;314:185–91.
23. Gallacher PD, Gilbert RE, Kanes G, et al. Outcome of meniscal repair prior compared with concurrent ACL reconstruction. Knee 2012;19(4):461–3.
24. Mesiha M, Zurakowski D, Soriano J, et al. Pathologic characteristics of the torn human meniscus. Am J Sports Med 2007;35:103–12.

25. Matsubara H, Okazaki K, Izawa T, et al. New suture method for radial tears of the meniscus: biomechanical analysis of cross-suture and double horizontal suture techniques using cyclic load testing. Am J Sports Med 2012;40(2):414–8.
26. Allaire R, Muriuki M, Gilbertson L, et al. Biomechanical consequences of a tear of the posterior root of the medial meniscus: similar to total meniscectomy. J Bone Joint Surg Am 2008;90(9):1922–31.
27. Noyes FR, Barber-Westin SD. Arthroscopic repair of meniscus tears extending into the avascular zone with or without anterior cruciate ligament reconstruction in patients 40 years of age and older. Arthroscopy 2000;16(8):822–9.
28. Bach BR, Dennis M, Balin J, et al. Arthroscopic meniscal repair: analysis of treatment failures. J Knee Surg 2005;18:278–84.
29. Grant JA, Wilde J, Miller BS, et al. Comparison of inside-out and all-inside techniques for the repair of isolated meniscal tears: a systematic review. Am J Sports Med 2012;40(2):459–68.
30. Abdelkafy A, Aigner N, Zada M, et al. Two to nineteen years follow-up of arthroscopic meniscal repair using the outside-in technique: a retrospective study. Arch Orthop Trauma Surg 2007;127(4):245–52.
31. Barrett GR, Treacy SH, Ruff CG. Preliminary results of the T-fix endoscopic meniscus repair technique in an anterior cruciate ligament reconstruction population. Arthroscopy 1997;13:218–23.
32. Escalas F, Quadras J, Caceres E, et al. T-Fix anchor sutures for arthroscopic meniscal repair. Knee Surg Sports Traumatol Arthrosc 1997;5:72–6.
33. Gill SS, Diduch DR. Outcomes after meniscal repair using the meniscus arrow in knees undergoing concurrent anterior cruciate ligament reconstruction. Arthroscopy 2002;18:569–77.
34. Lee GP, Diduch DR. Deteriorating outcomes after meniscal repair using the meniscus arrow in knees undergoing concurrent anterior cruciate ligament reconstruction: increased failure rate with long-term follow-up. Am J Sports Med 2005;33:1138–41.
35. Gifstad T, Grontvedt T, Drogset JO. Meniscal repair with Biofix arrows: results after 4.7 years' follow-up. Am J Sports Med 2007;35:71–4.
36. Haas AL, Schepsis AA, Hornstein J, et al. Meniscal repair using the FasT-Fix all-inside meniscal repair device. Arthroscopy 2005;21:167–75.
37. Quinby JS, Golish SR, Hart JA, et al. All-inside meniscal repair using a new flexible, tensionable device. Am J Sports Med 2006;34:1281–6.
38. Kohn D, Siebert W. Meniscus suture techniques: a comparative biomechanical cadaver study. Arthroscopy 1989;5:324–7.
39. Post WR, Akers SR, Kish V, et al. Load to failure of common meniscal repair techniques: effects of suture technique and suture material. Arthroscopy 1997;13:731–6.
40. Rimmer MG, Nawana NS, Keene GC, et al. Failure strengths of different meniscal suturing techniques. Arthroscopy 1995;11:146–50.
41. Wolf B, Rodeo S. Arthroscopic meniscus repair with suture: inside-out with fibrin clot. Sports Med Arthrosc Rev 2004;12:15–24.
42. Lambert E, Bonner K. Arthroscopic meniscus repair with sutures: outside-in. Sports Med Arthrosc Rev 2004;12:25–36.
43. Elkousy H, Higgins LD. Zone-specific inside-out meniscal repair: technical limitations of repair of posterior horns of medial and lateral menisci. Am J Orthop 2005;34(1):29–34.
44. Aldrich D, Anschuetz R, LoPresti C, et al. Pseudoaneurysm complicating knee arthroscopy. Arthroscopy 1995;11(2):229–30.

45. Jurist KA, Greene PW III, Shirkhoda A. Peroneal nerve dysfunction as a complication of lateral meniscus repair: a case report and anatomic dissection. Arthroscopy 1989;5(2):141–7.
46. Chen NC, Martin SD, Gill TJ. Risk to the lateral geniculate artery during arthroscopic lateral meniscal suture passage. Arthroscopy 2007;23(6):642–6.
47. Morgan CD. The "all-inside" meniscal repair. Arthroscopy 1991;7:120–5.
48. Calder SJ, Myers PT. Broken arrow: a complication of meniscal repair. Arthroscopy 1999;15(6):651–2.
49. Kumar A, Malhan K, Roberts SN. Chondral injury from bioabsorbable screws after meniscal repair. Arthroscopy 2001;17(8):34.
50. Barber FA, Herbert MA, Richards DP. Load to failure testing of new meniscal repair devices. Arthroscopy 2004;20:45–50.
51. Borden P, Nyland J, Caborn DN, et al. Biomechanical comparison of the FasT-Fix meniscal repair suture system with vertical mattress sutures and meniscus arrows. Am J Sports Med 2003;31:374–8.
52. Ochi M, Uchio Y, Okuda K, et al. Expression of cytokines after meniscal rasping to promote meniscal healing. Arthroscopy 2001;17(7):724–31.
53. Henning CE, Lynch MA, Yearout KM, et al. Arthroscopic meniscal repair using an exogenous fibrin clot. Clin Orthop 1990;252:64–72.
54. Becker R, Wirz D, Wolf C, et al. Measurement of meniscofemoral contact pressure after repair of bucket-handle tears with biodegradable implants. Arch Orthop Trauma Surg 2005;125(4):254–60.
55. Johal P, Williams A, Wragg P, et al. Tibio-femoral movement in the living knee: a study of weight bearing and non-weight bearing knee kinematics using 'interventional' MRI. J Biomech 2005;38(2):269–76.
56. Tienen TG, Buma P, Scholten JG, et al. Displacement of the medial meniscus within the passive motion characteristics of the human knee joint: an RSA study in human cadaver knees. Knee Surg Sports Traumatol Arthrosc 2005;13(4): 287–92.
57. Shelbourne KD, Patel DV, Adsit WS, et al. Rehabilitation after meniscal repair. Clin Sports Med 1996;15:595–612.
58. Barber FA. Accelerated rehabilitation for meniscus repairs. Arthroscopy 1994; 10(2):206–10.
59. Mariani PP, Santori N, Adriani E, et al. Accelerated rehabilitation after arthroscopic meniscal repair: a clinical and magnetic resonance imaging evaluation. Arthroscopy 1996;12:680–6.
60. Matava M. Meniscal allograft transplantation: a systematic review. Clin Orthop Relat Res 2007;455:142–57.
61. Graf K, Sekiya J, Wojtys E. Long-term results after combined medial meniscal allograft transplantation and anterior cruciate ligament reconstruction: minimum 8.5-year follow-up study. Arthroscopy 2004;20:129–40.
62. Garrett J, Stevenson R. Meniscal transplantation in the human knee: a preliminary report. Arthroscopy 1991;7:57–62.

Intra-articular Hip Disorders in the Military Population: Evaluation and Management

F. Winston Gwathmey Jr, MD*,
Warren R. Kadrmas, MD, MC, Col(s), USAF†

KEYWORDS

- Hip arthroscopy • Acetabular labral tear • Femoroacetabular impingement • Pincer
- Cam • Hip dysplasia

KEY POINTS

- Hip disorders are common in the military population given the physical demands and demographics.
- The at-risk hip joint (1) has abnormal morphology that leads to impingement during the arc of motion, and (2) is exposed to supraphysiologic stresses, either acute or chronic.
- Femoroacetabular impingement is a dynamic problem that it occurs because the hip is under stress from the activities to which it is exposed.
- Intra-articular damage may be acute, but is usually the result of the cumulative effects of repetitive abnormal contact between the ball and socket.
- Radiographic abnormalities around the hip are common and a systematic approach to hip dysfunction requires integration of components from the history, physical examination, imaging, and arthroscopic findings.
- Hip arthroscopy is a powerful emerging tool in the management of hip disorders.
- Recognizing and correcting the underlying bony problem is fundamental to successful treating hip disorders.

INTRODUCTION

The hip joint has received considerable attention recently as an evolving understanding of the pathoanatomy and injury factors inherent in the femoroacetabular articulation has prompted clinicians to recognize, evaluate, and treat hip dysfunction at younger ages and earlier in the disease process. Sparked in part by the work of Ganz and colleagues[1] promoting the concept of femoroacetabular impingement (FAI), the management paradigm for hip disease has shifted from reactively treating

Sports Medicine and Hip Arthroscopy, Department of Orthopaedic Surgery, University of Virginia Health System, 400 Ray C. Hunt Drive, Suite 330, Charlottesville, VA 22903, USA
† Deceased.
* Corresponding author.
E-mail address: fwg7d@virginia.edu

Clin Sports Med 33 (2014) 655–674
http://dx.doi.org/10.1016/j.csm.2014.06.013
0278-5919/14/$ – see front matter © 2014 Elsevier Inc. All rights reserved.
sportsmed.theclinics.com

the consequences of arthritis in advanced age toward recognizing and preemptively addressing the factors that lead to hip damage and degeneration in younger patients. The proliferation of hip arthroscopy has further expanded understanding of hip disease and has provided innovative treatment options.

The femoroacetabular articulation is a highly congruent ball and socket joint deep within the body that generally does not lend itself to damage or injury under normal circumstances with routine activity, when the morphology is normal. Unlike the more peripheral joints of the upper and lower extremity that are vulnerable to high external forces and moment arms, the hip joint is protected by a secure connection to the pelvis that limits extremes of motion and a thick soft tissue envelope that softens impact. Two primary factors should therefore be considered when evaluating the injured hip joint: the shape of the joint and the stress on the joint.

The at-risk hip joint is (1) has underlying skeletal morphology that leads to abnormal mechanics between the ball and socket; and/or (2) is exposed to supraphysiologic stress, either acute or chronic. These two factors are not mutually exclusively, and most patients who present with hip complaints have components of both. The magnitude of damage correlates with the severity of the structural incongruity and the amount of activity-related stress on the joint. Those patients who routinely expose the hip to greater forces or higher cumulative stress may overwhelm normal anatomy, whereas those patients with greater femoroacetabular deformity may experience symptoms earlier in life with less cumulative stress.

The military population is particularly at risk for hip disorders given the demographics and demands inherent this population.[2] Abnormal femoroacetabular morphology, especially cam deformity, is commonly seen in the young, athletic men who make up much of the military population.[3–6] High levels of athletic activity during skeletal development may contribute to abnormal morphology.[7,8] The physical demands of military training and active duty are similar to those of elite athletics and military personnel are susceptible to acute injuries to the hip as well as overuse conditions.[9,10] Joint reactive forces within the hip may exceed 5 times body weight during rigorous athletic activity.[11–13] Higher overall activity levels within the military population have been associated with higher incidence rates of hip osteoarthritis compared with the general population.[14]

ANATOMY

The skeletal junction between the pelvis and leg is the femoroacetabular articulation. Almost all motion at this diarthroidal joint is rotational, the limits of which are conferred by the configuration of the ball within the socket and the surrounding ligamentous structures. The articular surfaces of the hip joint are highly congruent with intrinsic stability provided by a deep acetabular vault that covers 170° of the femoral head.[15,16]

A fibrocartilaginous labrum that runs circumferentially around the acetabular rim augments hip stability, deepening the socket by as much as 20%.[15,17–19] Conforming to the perimeter of the femoral head through the arc of motion, the labrum has numerous functions including maintenance of negative intra-articular pressure, regulation of the intra-articular hydrostatic synovial fluid pressure, and even distribution of forces across the joint. Further stability is provided by a thick, fibrous joint capsule that contains the strongest ligaments in the body.[19,20]

Functioning synchronously, the hip joints form the static and dynamic foundation on which the upper body is positioned and moves over the legs. Through the complex integration of dynamic and static stabilizers around the multiaxial ball and socket joint, the normally functioning hip joints effortlessly support the body and maintain pelvic and spinal balance during activity. The free rotational mobility of the joint necessitates collaboration of multiple muscle groups to control and stabilize motion.

Twenty-four muscles cross the hip joint, some of which are the largest and most powerful in the body. The same muscles that maintain the intricate equilibrium of lumbopelvic stabilization are also capable of initiating the explosive forces of jumping and running. Disorders within the hip joint may disrupt this delicate equilibrium and lead to secondary soft tissue problems and injuries around the pelvis.

PATHOPHYSIOLOGY

The bony anatomy of the hip joint is highly variable and has implications for the pathophysiology of hip joint dysfunction.[21,22] As the skeleton grows, the acetabulum and femoral head form together as unit, and normal development requires a delicate, genetically mediated balance between the converging triradiate cartilages of the acetabular fossa and the well-centered femoral head.[23] Genetic and/or developmental factors may result in an articulation that is not biomechanically optimized for the daily demands imposed on the joint. External forces on the proximal femoral physes of the growing skeleton from rigorous activity during adolescence may further contribute to deformities that detrimentally affect the femoroacetabular articulation.[7,24]

In the mature skeleton, pathologic hip joint mechanics are generally within a continuum between undercoverage (dysplasia) and overcoverage (FAI).[25] The cumulative effect of the stress on the joint resulting from the pathologic mechanics leads to secondary damage to the cartilage, labrum, and joint capsule with progressive joint dysfunction and degeneration.

Developmental Dysplasia

Developmental dysplasia of the hip occurs when the hip joint does not properly form and leads to a shallow acetabular socket with variable deformity of the proximal femur. Present in approximately 1% of the population and most common in women, hip dysplasia represents a range of abnormalities that ranges from subtle radiographic findings to subluxation or frank dislocation.[26] The nonconcentric force distribution and subtle instability that underlie the dysplastic hip joint lead to eccentric cartilage wear and labral hypertrophy.[27-29]

Moderate to severe cases are commonly diagnosed and treated in infancy or early childhood.[26,30] In many cases of mild dysplasia, increased hip mobility and flexibility are the only objective physical examination findings and patients may otherwise be asymptomatic. Strain on dynamic secondary stabilizers may contribute to extraarticular conditions such as iliopsoas disorders or bursitis, and may produce the symptoms with which the dysplastic patient first presents. Intra-articular symptoms develop insidiously with secondary labral damage to the labrum or joint degeneration.

Femoroacetabular Impingement

The skeletal morphology that underlies FAI causes abnormal contact between the proximal femur and acetabulum during the physiologic arc of motion.[25,31] This contact impedes terminal motion of the ball within the socket at certain leg positions. The deformity may be present on the acetabular side (pincer impingement), femoral side (cam impingement), or both.

Vital soft tissue structures may become trapped between the two hard bony surfaces leading to injury, inflammation, and progressive joint degeneration. Varying degrees of injury to the joint occurs with acute forceful mechanisms or cumulative damage and is related to the structural abnormality and the magnitude and frequency of the stress. A mild deformity that is well tolerated by an average person may cause significant damage and dysfunction in someone who places rigorous demands on the joint, such as a military recruit.

Pincer

Pincer impingement occurs when acetabular overcoverage of the femoral head leads to premature contact between the acetabular rim and femoral neck (**Fig. 1**). Structural causes of pincer impingement include acetabular rim abnormalities, acetabular retroversion, and coxa profunda or protrusio. Anterior inferior iliac spine prominence may also create a pincer-type mechanism. Labral calcification or ossification may cause acquired pincer impingement.[32,33]

The pathologic deformity is usually located anteriorly in the joint and creates problems with hip flexion and internal rotation. As the femoral neck collides with rim, the labrum is pinched between the bony structures. Although a single forceful event may create a labral tear in this setting, the labral damage typically occurs more insidiously with repetitive trauma. Labral bruising, interstitial tearing, and/or fraying may be seen in cases of long-standing pincer impingement, with detachment occurring later in the disease process. Contre-coup cartilage and labral damage in the posterior joint

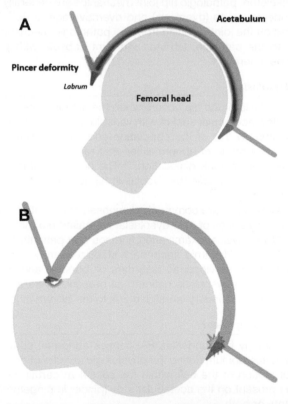

Fig. 1. (*A*) Pincer impingement results from an overhanging acetabular rim that impedes terminal hip flexion. (*B*) With increasing hip flexion, the femoral neck collides with the pincer deformity causing damage to the labrum. Repetitive impingement results in cumulative damage and tearing. The femoral head may also lever out of the socket causing contre-coup chondral damage to the posterior acetabulum.

may occur when the femoral head is levered out of the socket by the pincer mechanism and collides with the posterior wall of the acetabulum.[22]

Cam

Cam impingement results from a femoral-sided deformity in which a misshapen femoral head or prominence of the femoral head-neck junction creates an incongruity between the ball and socket at certain hip positions (**Fig. 2**). As suggested by the term cam, which refers to a machinery mechanism in which a rotating eccentric wheel or cylinder produces a reciprocating motion within the machine, cam impingement of the hip results when the eccentric portion of the femoral ball enters the acetabular socket. The round socket cannot accommodate the out-of-round portion of the femoral head and a mechanical conflict occurs between the two surfaces. Potential

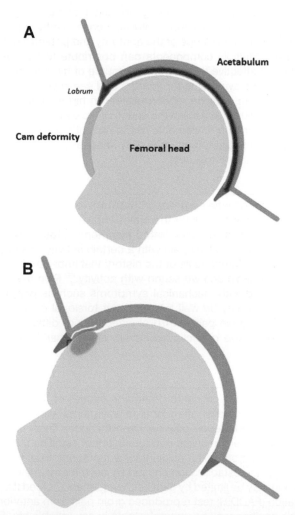

Fig. 2. (*A*) Cam impingement occurs with a loss of femoral head sphericity that creates a mechanical mismatch between the ball and socket. (*B*) With increasing flexion, the cam deformity engages the acetabular socket causing shear damage to the articular cartilage and disruption of the chondrolabral junction.

causes include asymmetrical closure of the capital femoral epiphysis, a focal bony prominence of the femoral head-neck junction, slipped capital-femoral epiphysis or physeal fracture, or osteophyte. There is increasing evidence that heavy athletic activity during adolescence may increase the risk for cam deformity.[8,34–36]

The pathologic deformity of cam impingement is most commonly located anteriorly or superolaterally on the femur and creates problems with hip flexion, adduction, and internal rotation.[31] As the prominence on the femoral head engages the acetabular vault, shear forces are exerted on the articular cartilage and chondrolabral junction. Damage occurs with repetitive impingement and focal cartilage delamination and failure of the chondrolabral junction may occur with long-standing impingement.

EVALUATION OF THE HIP

There is no single clinical finding or imaging modality that can definitively diagnose a hip condition or injury. Evaluation of the painful hip consequently requires a systematic approach and an intricate knowledge of the anatomy and potential pathologic entities around the hip joint. Multiple components can contribute to hip dysfunction, each requiring attention for effective treatment. The source of hip pain can be elusive and patients may experience symptoms for months and see several physicians before a cause is recognized.[37] In addition, abnormalities on hip imaging are common and do not necessarily definitively establish the cause of hip dysfunction.[6,38,39] Successful diagnosis requires integration of elements of the patient's history, physical examination, plain imaging, computed tomography (CT), magnetic resonance imaging (MRI), diagnostic injections, and arthroscopy.

History

The patient history provides the essential groundwork for the evaluation of the painful hip. Important considerations include the onset and duration of symptoms, exacerbating positions or activities, and associated symptoms. Most patients do not recall a specific event but associate their pain with a certain activity or a change in training exercises or intensity.[37] Components of the history that implicate the hip joint include pain localizable to the groin and worsened with activity.[40] Pain may be sharp or dull and may be associated with mechanical symptoms such as popping or catching. Straight-plane activities may be well tolerated but torsional or pivoting movements elicit discomfort. Deep groin pain with prolonged sitting, difficult putting on socks and shoes, and progressive pain climbing stairs are hallmarks of intra-articular hip disorders.[4]

Physical Examination

An organized examination is critical to determine causes of the painful hip. Patients with intra-articular hip problems often localize symptoms with the C sign, in which they cup the lateral hip and report pain between the index finger and thumb.[40,41] An antalgic gait may be present in cases of acute injury or significant hip joint irritability. Gait abnormalities may also reflect involuntary adaptations to offload a problematic hip joint or lumbopelvic destabilization caused by asymmetry in the hip musculature. Hip range of motion may be limited by pain or impingement. Forced flexion, adduction, and internal rotation (FADDIR) test reproduces groin pain from anterior labral tears or FAI, although this position may be uncomfortable in any irritable hip. Flexion, abduction and external rotation (FABER) test may elicit anterior or anterolateral pain in cases of impingement. The hip flexors, adductors, and abductors, as well as lower abdominal muscles, should be evaluated for tenderness, tightness, and/or weakness to identify compensatory conditions that may be contributing to the overall dysfunction of the hip.

Imaging

Plain radiographs are fundamental to diagnosing and understanding hip disorders. A well-centered anteroposterior (AP) pelvis and lateral view of the affected hip shows the skeletal morphology that underlies the dysfunctional hip. A false-profile view of the acetabulum is also helpful to determine anterior coverage as well as anterosuperior joint space. Skeletal morphologic variations that predispose to hip dysfunction should be carefully assessed. In addition, other conditions should be considered such as stress reactions or fractures, degenerative joint disease, and disorders involving the pubic symphysis, sacroiliac joints, and lumbar spine. Loss of joint space, sclerosis, subchondral cystic formation, and osteophytes suggest osteoarthritis and portend a less favorable prognosis.

FAI morphology is commonly seen on radiographs of patients with hip pain.[42] On the acetabular side, features of pincer impingement include increased lateral center-edge angle, crossover sign, ischial spine sign, and coxa profunda or protrusio (**Fig. 3**).[43,44] The false-profile view is helpful to show abnormalities of the anterior inferior iliac spine, which predispose to pincer-type impingement. Secondary changes on the femoral neck from repetitive abutment, such as herniation pits, may also be seen on plain radiographs. Cam impingement is suggested by loss of femoral head/neck offset and an increased alpha angle (**Fig. 4**).[43] Cam deformities are frequently located anteriorly on the femoral neck and are best seen on a lateral radiograph of the hip.[44]

Similar or identical morphology may be present on the contralateral asymptomatic side and does not necessarily reflect a problem. FAI morphology is commonly seen in asymptomatic patients, and abnormal radiographs alone are not sufficient to diagnose FAI. In one study of 95 asymptomatic elite soccer players, radiographic findings meeting criteria of FAI were seen in 72% of male and 50% of female players.[6] However, special attention should be paid to onset of symptoms in previously asymptomatic patients with radiographic findings consistent with impingement because these patients may benefit from earlier surgical correction to possibly prevent irreversible secondary damage.[44]

Radiographs should be scrutinized for features of potential hip dysplasia because this may affect the treatment algorithm. Dysplasia is characterized by shallow

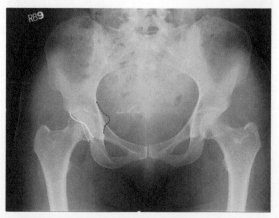

Fig. 3. Radiographic features of pincer impingement include increased lateral and/or anterior center-edge angle, crossover sign, and ischial spine sign as shown on this AP radiograph.

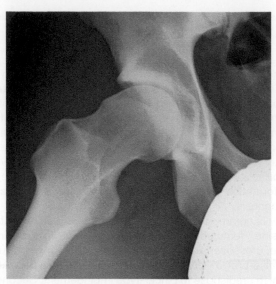

Fig. 4. Loss of femoral head sphericity and head-neck offset, as seen on this 45° Dunn lateral radiograph, are radiographic features of cam impingement.

acetabular sockets with femoral head undercoverage and should be considered if there is a center-edge angle of less than 20° to 25° laterally and/or anteriorly (**Fig. 5**).[32] An up-sloping sourcil with a Tonnis angle of greater than 10 is also consistent with hip dysplasia.

Cross-sectional imaging
The complex three-dimensional (3D) anatomy of the femoroacetabular articulation is best shown by cross-sectional imaging. MRI is the most commonly used test to diagnose intra-articular hip disorders because it provides outstanding definition of the labrum and soft tissue structures around the hip (**Fig. 6**).[45,46] MRI may also show secondary findings such as intraosseous and soft tissue edema, paralabral and

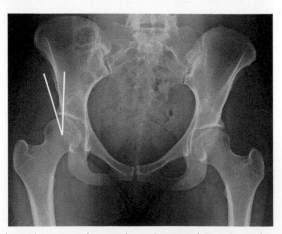

Fig. 5. Decreased lateral center-edge angle or increased Tonnis angle as seen on this AP pelvis radiograph are radiographic markers of acetabular dysplasia.

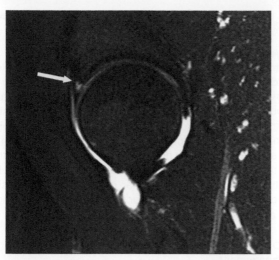

Fig. 6. Magnetic resonance arthrogram of an anterior labral tear (*arrow*) showing signal penetrating the chondrolabral junction.

subchondral cysts, and effusions. The addition of intra-articular contrast with magnetic resonance (MR) arthrography improves sensitivity and specificity, in particular for labral disorders.

CT is the modality of choice to fully characterize bony morphology.[32,47–49] Although plain radiography can only provide a two-dimensional representation of the hip and MRI is limited in its ability to clearly delineate bony architecture, CT delivers precise images of the osseous structures and can be reformatted to analyze complex deformities in multiple dimensions (**Fig. 7**). In addition, manipulation of 3D reconstructions allows the surgeon to gain considerable insight into the relationship between the

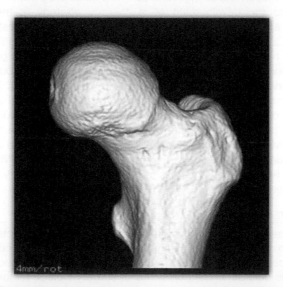

Fig. 7. 3D CT of the proximal femur shows the 3D anatomy of the cam deformity.

acetabulum and proximal femur. CT has been used more as surgeons increasingly consider the bony morphology that underlies hip disorders.

Intra-articular injection

Image-guided intra-articular injection of local anesthetic is a valuable diagnostic tool to elucidate hip disorders.[46,50] The anatomic region around the hip joint is complex and the differential diagnosis for pain in this region is broad. Localizing pain to an intra-articular source is essential to establishing an effective treatment algorithm. Concomitant extra-articular disorders often obscure the clinical picture and eliminating pain emanating from the joint allows accurate assessment of the contribution of extra-articular sources. Minimal or no anesthetic response to an intra-articular injection should raise the index of suspicion for an alternative diagnosis, whereas a positive response strongly suggests an intra-articular disorder.[46] The injection may be performed in conjunction with an arthrogram for MR or CT or as a diagnostic/therapeutic preparation with a corticosteroid.

MANAGEMENT OF INTRA-ARTICULAR HIP DISORDERS
Nonoperative Management

The treatment algorithm for most intra-articular hip disorders starts with a trial of conservative treatment.[51,52] Early goals include controlling pain and reducing inflammation. The irritable hip alters the surrounding pelvic biomechanics as the patient attempts to offload the joint. This alteration produces pathologic gait accommodations and secondary problems within the dynamic stabilizers around the hip. Additional strain occurs at adjacent joints in the pelvis and the lumbar spine as they compensate for the motion lost at the hip joint.[53] Addressing pain and inflammation within the hip promotes more efficient and successful normalization of motion and gait. Rest, activity modification, oral antiinflammatories, and intra-articular corticosteroid injections are effective options.

Once the joint is calmed down, physical therapy is instituted to restore function and optimize pelvic mechanics. A functional assessment may be useful to identify asymmetry in range of motion and strength and can help guide progression through the protocol. Central to the development of a therapy strategy is the concept that impingement is a dynamic problem. The anatomy of the joint must be considered when designing a protocol because some limitation of range of motion may be expected with FAI morphology. Therapy should focus on restoring a pain-free physiologic arc of motion within the bony constraints of the femoroacetabular morphology. Strength deficiencies should be addressed and gait normalized. Manual therapy and modalities may be integrated to alleviate soft tissue discomfort and tightness.

The ultimate goal of conservative management is to establish durable pelvic mechanics that will protect the hip joint from injury throughout routine as well as strenuous activities. Much of this involves neuromuscular training and learning how to avoid the positions that provoke impingement. The patient's activity requirements should be considered so that strategies to prevent further joint injury can be incorporated into the therapy program.

Hip Arthroscopy

Surgery should be considered for symptomatic patients with suspected intra-articular disorders that do not respond to conservative treatment. Common indications include symptomatic acetabular labral tears, chondral injuries, loose bodies, FAI, and ligamentum teres disorders. The objectives of surgery include removing mechanical or structural elements contributing to symptoms and addressing or repairing intra-articular damage that has occurred. In patients with FAI, correcting the bony impingement is essential to preventing further secondary damage and may help slow or prevent development of arthritis.

Although open procedures such as surgical dislocation and mini–open anterior approaches have been used to address intra-articular hip disorders, hip arthroscopy has emerged as a powerful diagnostic and therapeutic tool that is well suited to treating intra-articular disorders in the active military population.[2] In the past it has lagged behind arthroscopy of the knee and shoulder because of inherent anatomic constraints and technological obstacles, but hip arthroscopy has recently increased in use, fueled by expanding indications and technical advances.[54,55] It is now the most popular technique for treatment of most athletic hip injuries.[56,57]

Advantages of hip arthroscopy include outstanding visualization and documentation of intra-articular disorders and the capability to perform intricate repairs and bony corrections through a minimally invasive, soft tissue–sparing procedure. Larger bony corrections and osteotomies, in particular on the acetabular side, are difficult with arthroscopy and necessitate an open procedure. Low complication rates have been reported for hip arthroscopy and include traction-related and/or compression-related neurapraxias to the pudendal, sciatic, and/or femoral nerves; injury to the lateral femoral cutaneous nerve; compressive damage to the perineum or foot; iatrogenic damage to the labrum or cartilage; instrument breakage within the joint; iatrogenic instability; heterotopic ossification; and fluid extravasation into the thigh or abdomen.[58–60] However, hip arthroscopy is associated with a steep learning curve, and special training and experience are needed to limit complication risk.[61]

Technique

Hip arthroscopy is performed in the supine or lateral position.[62,63] Essential to successful hip arthroscopy is the ability to safely pull the femoral head out of the acetabular socket, and a number of operating tables have been developed to allow this.[64] General anesthesia with complete muscle paralysis and approximately 9 to 23 kg (25 to 50 pounds) of traction are required to effectively distract the joint the 8 to 10 mm needed to instrument within the joint.[65,66] Traction should be limited to less than 2 hours.[67] For optimal visualization and instrumentation within the joint, both the 70° and 30° arthroscopes are needed as well as specialized extralength instruments. Fluoroscopy is used throughout the procedure to guide portal placement and direct bony correction.

Two arthroscopic spaces within the hip joint have been described: the central compartment and the peripheral compartment.[68] The central compartment is the space within the acetabular vault between the ball and socket and requires traction for access. Disorders addressed in the central compartment include labral tears, chondral damage on the femoral head and within the acetabulum, ligamentum teres tears, loose bodies, iliopsoas disorders, pincer deformities, and os acetabuli.

The peripheral compartment comprising the intra-articular space within the capsule but outside the femoroacetabular articulation is accessed with the hip out of traction and in some degree of flexion to relax the anterior joint capsule. The most common procedure in the peripheral compartment is correction of cam deformity. Other peripheral compartment procedures include loose body removal, synovectomy, iliopsoas release, and capsular plication or repair. Dynamic assessment of the labral seal and the mechanics of the femoral head within the acetabulum with hip range of motion may also be performed in the peripheral compartment.

The landmarks used to establish portals include the anterior superior iliac spine (ASIS) and the greater trochanter. The safe zone for hip arthroscopy is the space lateral and distal to the intersection of the longitudinal line drawn distally from the ASIS and a transverse line drawn anteriorly from the greater trochanter.[69,70] The standard initial viewing portal for hip arthroscopy is the anterolateral portal established just anterior to the tip of the greater trochanter. Several anterior working portals have been described as well as accessory proximal and distal portals.[70]

Labral tears

Acetabular labral tears are among the most common indications for hip arthroscopy because they may produce the mechanical symptoms responsible for presentation (**Fig. 8**).[66,71] Arthroscopic debridement or repair of the labrum with suture anchors have been described as strategies to relieve pain by eliminating the unstable flap responsible for hip discomfort.[66,71,72] There is increasing evidence that the acetabular labrum plays a vital role in the mechanics of the femoroacetabular articulation and it should be preserved.[18,73–76] It is also important to recall that labral tears rarely occur in the absence of bony abnormalities, and repairing the labrum without correcting the mechanical environment contributing to the tear may not provide a lasting fix.[21,66,77,78]

Cartilage damage

Chondral damage to the acetabulum and/or femoral head may be addressed arthroscopically. Cartilage damage may occur from acute injury such a lateral impact injury but more commonly from chronic mechanical mismatch from FAI or dysplasia.[22,79] Cartilage has limited ability to heal and loose chondral flaps may be debrided arthroscopically. Microfracture has been used with some success for full-thickness focal defects.[80,81] Other cartilage repair/restoration techniques such as autologous chondrocyte implantation and osteochondral allografting have been described but are used less frequently in the hip than in other joints.[82] As with labral repair, correcting the bony morphology contributing to the secondary damage is essential to treatment of hip articular cartilage lesions.

FAI

The evolving understanding of the mechanics underlying FAI has promoted the transformation of hip arthroscopy from primarily a soft tissue procedure to largely a bony

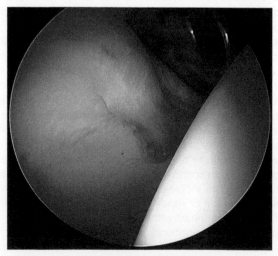

Fig. 8. Arthroscopic appearance of an anterior labral tear.

procedure. Successful management of secondary cartilage and labral damage requires correction of the underlying impingement pattern. Effective surgical osteoplasty can improve range of motion and eliminate the recurrent mechanical collision from FAI.[3] Systematic preoperative evaluation with examination and imaging is fundamental to treating FAI. Reformatted CT scan with 3D reconstruction is increasingly used to template bony correction, and effective execution of the surgical correction is guided by intraoperative fluoroscopy.[49,81,83,84]

Correction of pincer deformity is performed by trimming the prominent rim of acetabular bone that is responsible for impingement. Often the labrum in the region of pincer impingement is contused or torn as it is caught between the overhanging rim and the femoral neck, and this finding helps to localize the region of impingement.[22,79,85] To access the pincer deformity, the capsular aspect of the labrum is dissected from the bony rim or alternatively the labrum can be completely detached. A high-speed burr is used to recess the acetabular rim to decompress the area of impingement. Intraoperative fluoroscopy helps to localize position on the rim and to monitor for correction of the crossover sign. Traction may be released during pincer correction to verify smooth contour and adequate decompression. After pincer correction, the labrum is refixed to the rim acetabular rim with suture anchors. Loose, devitalized labral fragments may be debrided.

Cam impingement has been labeled the silent killer of the hip because of the detrimental impact of the deformity on the acetabular cartilage.[86] Long-standing cam impingement generates failure of the chondrolabral junction and delamination of the articular cartilage (**Fig. 9**).[31,87,88] Although the secondary damage is typically seen in the central compartment, the disorder is accessed in the peripheral compartment. However, the locations and pattern of acetabular chondral damage can help localize the prominence in the femoral neck. Correction of cam impingement involves using a high-speed burr to reshape the femoral head-neck junction (**Fig. 10**). The leg is rotated to access the far medial and far lateral aspects of the deformity and the limits of correction are regulated by the medial and lateral synovial folds. Judicious use of

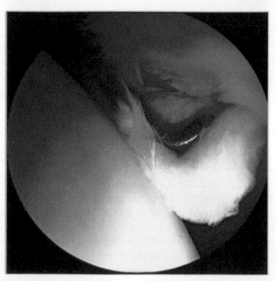

Fig. 9. Long-standing cam impingement can cause chondral delamination with repetitive shear stress across the articular cartilage.

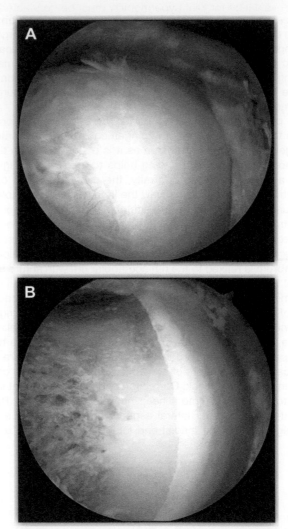

Fig. 10. (*A*) Arthroscopic appearance of a cam deformity of the proximal femur. (*B*) A high-speed burr is used to reshape the cam deformity to decompress the zone of impingement.

fluoroscopy during cam decompression is recommended to ensure appropriate correction.[84]

Rehabilitation

The minimally invasive approach of hip arthroscopy leaves little external evidence of how much work was performed inside the joint and patients should be reminded that they have undergone a major procedure. Early goals of rehabilitation include decreasing edema and inflammation while maintaining hip mobility with an emphasis on protecting the repair. Early therapy is recommended to facilitate efficient recovery of function. Surgeons may implement weight-bearing restrictions, range-of-motion restrictions, and/or bracing to limit the stress on the cartilage, labral, or capsular repair as well as on the bony correction. Some surgeons use continuous passive motion to prevent adhesion formation. Late goals of rehabilitation include normalizing range of motion and gait and restoring strength around the hip with the ultimate goal of returning to a previous level of sport or activity. It generally takes at least 3 to 6 months for return to full activity depending on the procedure performed.

SUMMARY

The physical demands of the military expose the hip to extreme forces and stresses and generate a high incidence of hip disorders within this population. Fundamental to the pathophysiology of hip injuries is the underlying anatomy of the joint because problematic femoroacetabular mechanics predispose to injury. FAI is increasingly recognized as the underlying cause of hip disorders and should be considered when assessing a patient with hip complaints. Young, male patients are at increased risk of FAI, especially cam impingement, and high levels of athletic activity during skeletal growth may contribute to the development of cam morphology. A complete evaluation requires a careful history and physical examination combined with multiple imaging modalities. Conservative treatment is indicated for acute hip injury to allow alleviation of inflammation and restoration of normal gait and range of motion. Surgery should be considered for refractory dysfunction, mechanical symptoms, or significant deformities. Arthroscopy has revolutionized the treatment of hip injuries in young, active patients, and is likely to continue to expand in use.

REFERENCES

1. Ganz R, Parvizi J, Beck M, et al. Femoroacetabular impingement: a cause for osteoarthritis of the hip. Clin Orthop Relat Res 2003;(417):112–20. http://dx.doi.org/10.1097/01.blo.0000096804.78689.c2.
2. Murphy KP, Freedman BA, Giuliani JG. Arthroscopic management of intra-articular hip disorders in active-duty military patients. Oper Tech Sports Med 2005;13(3):143–9. http://dx.doi.org/10.1053/j.otsm.2005.10.009.
3. Bedi A, Dolan M, Hetsroni I, et al. Surgical treatment of femoroacetabular impingement improves hip kinematics: a computer-assisted model. Am J Sports Med 2011;39(Suppl):43S–9S. http://dx.doi.org/10.1177/0363546511414635.
4. Clohisy JC, Knaus ER, Hunt DM, et al. Clinical presentation of patients with symptomatic anterior hip impingement. Clin Orthop Relat Res 2009;467(3): 638–44. http://dx.doi.org/10.1007/s11999-008-0680-y.
5. Hack K, Di Primio G, Rakhra K, et al. Prevalence of cam-type femoroacetabular impingement morphology in asymptomatic volunteers. J Bone Joint Surg Am 2010;92(14):2436–44. http://dx.doi.org/10.2106/JBJS.J.01280.
6. Gerhardt MB, Romero AA, Silvers HJ, et al. The prevalence of radiographic hip abnormalities in elite soccer players. Am J Sports Med 2012;40(3):584–8. http://dx.doi.org/10.1177/0363546511432711.
7. Siebenrock KA, Behning A, Mamisch TC, et al. Growth plate alteration precedes cam-type deformity in elite basketball players. Clin Orthop Relat Res 2013; 471(4):1084–91. http://dx.doi.org/10.1007/s11999-012-2740-6.
8. Kienle KP, Keck J, Werlen S, et al. Femoral morphology and epiphyseal growth plate changes of the hip during maturation: MR assessments in a 1-year follow-up on a cross-sectional asymptomatic cohort in the age range of 9-17 years. Skeletal Radiol 2012;41(11):1381–90. http://dx.doi.org/10.1007/s00256-012-1358-9.
9. Kaufman KR, Brodine S, Shaffer R. Military training-related injuries: surveillance, research, and prevention. Am J Prev Med 2000;18(Suppl 3):54–63. Available at: http://www.ncbi.nlm.nih.gov/pubmed/10736541. Accessed June 3, 2014.

10. Armed Forces Health Surveillance Center (AFHSC). Injuries associated with combat sports, active component, U.S. Armed Forces, 2010-2013. MSMR 2014;21(5):16–8. Available at: http://www.ncbi.nlm.nih.gov/pubmed/24885879. Accessed June 3, 2014.

11. Shindle MK, Ranawat AS, Kelly BT. Diagnosis and management of traumatic and atraumatic hip instability in the athletic patient. Clin Sports Med 2006; 25(2):309–26. http://dx.doi.org/10.1016/j.csm.2005.12.003, ix–x.

12. Byrne DP, Mulhall KJ, Baker JF. Anatomy & biomechanics of the hip. Open Sports Med J 2010;4:51–7.

13. Stal DN, Ferguson S, Incavo SJ, et al. Biomechanics of the natural hip joint. In: Berry DJ, Lieberman JR, editors. Surgery of the hip. Philadelphia: Elsevier; 2013. p. 2–18. http://dx.doi.org/10.1016/B978-0-443-06991-8.00001-2.

14. Scher DL, Belmont PJ, Mountcastle S, et al. The incidence of primary hip osteoarthritis in active duty US military servicemembers. Arthritis Rheum 2009;61(4): 468–75. http://dx.doi.org/10.1002/art.24429.

15. Shu B, Safran MR. Hip instability: anatomic and clinical considerations of traumatic and atraumatic instability. Clin Sports Med 2011;30(2):349–67. http://dx. doi.org/10.1016/j.csm.2010.12.008.

16. Boykin RE, Anz AW, Bushnell BD, et al. Hip instability. J Am Acad Orthop Surg 2011;19(6):340–9. Available at: http://www.ncbi.nlm.nih.gov/pubmed/21628645. Accessed January 27, 2013.

17. Kelly BT, Shapiro GS, Digiovanni CW, et al. Vascularity of the hip labrum: a cadaveric investigation. Arthroscopy 2005;21(1):3–11. http://dx.doi.org/10. 1016/j.arthro.2004.09.016.

18. Crawford MJ, Dy CJ, Alexander JW, et al. The 2007 Frank Stinchfield Award. The biomechanics of the hip labrum and the stability of the hip. Clin Orthop Relat Res 2007;465(465):16–22. http://dx.doi.org/10.1097/BLO.0b013e31815b181f.

19. Myers CA, Register BC, Lertwanich P, et al. Role of the acetabular labrum and the iliofemoral ligament in hip stability: an in vitro biplane fluoroscopy study. Am J Sports Med 2011;39(Suppl):85S–91S. http://dx.doi.org/10.1177/0363546511412161.

20. Telleria JJ, Lindsey DP, Giori NJ, et al. An anatomic arthroscopic description of the hip capsular ligaments for the hip arthroscopist. Arthroscopy 2011;27(5): 628–36. http://dx.doi.org/10.1016/j.arthro.2011.01.007.

21. Wenger DE, Kendell KR, Miner MR, et al. Acetabular labral tears rarely occur in the absence of bony abnormalities. Clin Orthop Relat Res 2004;426(426): 145–50. http://dx.doi.org/10.1097/01.blo.0000136903.01368.20.

22. Beck M, Kalhor M, Leunig M, et al. Hip morphology influences the pattern of damage to the acetabular cartilage: femoroacetabular impingement as a cause of early osteoarthritis of the hip. J Bone Joint Surg Br 2005;87(7):1012–8. http:// dx.doi.org/10.1302/0301-620X.87B7.15203.

23. Weinstein SL. Natural history of congenital hip dislocation (CDH) and hip dysplasia. Clin Orthop Relat Res 1987;(225):62–76. Available at: http://www. ncbi.nlm.nih.gov/pubmed/3315382. Accessed June 3, 2014.

24. Siebenrock KA, Schwab JM. The cam-type deformity–what is it: SCFE, osteophyte, or a new disease? J Pediatr Orthop 2013;33(Suppl 1):S121–5. http:// dx.doi.org/10.1097/BPO.0b013e3182771782.

25. Bedi A, Kelly BT. Femoroacetabular impingement. J Bone Joint Surg Am 2013; 95(1):82–92. http://dx.doi.org/10.2106/JBJS.K.01219.

26. Guille JT, Pizzutillo PD, MacEwen GD. Development dysplasia of the hip from birth to six months. J Am Acad Orthop Surg 2000;8(4):232–42. Available at: http://www.ncbi.nlm.nih.gov/pubmed/10951112. Accessed June 3, 2014.

27. Byrd JW, Jones KS. Hip arthroscopy in the presence of dysplasia. Arthroscopy 2003;19(10):1055–60. http://dx.doi.org/10.1016/j.arthro.2003.10.010.
28. Fujii M, Nakashima Y, Jingushi S, et al. Intraarticular findings in symptomatic developmental dysplasia of the hip. J Pediatr Orthop 2009;29(1):9–13. http://dx.doi.org/10.1097/BPO.0b013e318190a0be.
29. Bowman KF, Fox J, Sekiya JK. A clinically relevant review of hip biomechanics. Arthroscopy 2010;26(8):1118–29. http://dx.doi.org/10.1016/j.arthro.2010.01.027.
30. Gillingham B, Sanchez AA, Wenger DR. Pelvic osteotomies for the treatment of hip dysplasia in children and young adults. J Am Acad Orthop Surg 1999;7(5): 325–37. Available at: http://171.66.123.206/content/7/5/325.short. Accessed January 27, 2013.
31. Bedi A, Dolan M, Leunig M, et al. Static and dynamic mechanical causes of hip pain. Arthroscopy 2011;27(2):235–51. http://dx.doi.org/10.1016/j.arthro.2010.07.022.
32. Lynch TS, Terry MA, Bedi A, et al. Hip arthroscopic surgery: patient evaluation, current indications, and outcomes. Am J Sports Med 2013;41(5):1174–89. http://dx.doi.org/10.1177/0363546513476281.
33. Cooke WR, Gill HS, Murray DW, et al. Discrete mineralisation of the acetabular labrum: a novel marker of femoroacetabular impingement? Br J Radiol 2013; 86(1021):20120182. http://dx.doi.org/10.1259/bjr.20120182.
34. Siebenrock KA, Kaschka I, Frauchiger L, et al. Prevalence of cam-type deformity and hip pain in elite ice hockey players before and after the end of growth. Am J Sports Med 2013;41(10):2308–13. http://dx.doi.org/10.1177/0363546513497564.
35. Philippon MJ, Ho CP, Briggs KK, et al. Prevalence of increased alpha angles as a measure of cam-type femoroacetabular impingement in youth ice hockey players. Am J Sports Med 2013;41:1357–62. http://dx.doi.org/10.1177/0363546513483448.
36. Carsen S, Moroz PJ, Rakhra K, et al. The Otto Aufranc Award. On the etiology of the cam deformity: a cross-sectional pediatric MRI study. Clin Orthop Relat Res 2014;472:430–6. http://dx.doi.org/10.1007/s11999-013-2990-y.
37. Burnett RS, Della Rocca GJ, Prather H, et al. Clinical presentation of patients with tears of the acetabular labrum. J Bone Joint Surg Am 2006;88(7): 1448–57. http://dx.doi.org/10.2106/JBJS.D.02806.
38. Register B, Pennock AT, Ho CP, et al. Prevalence of abnormal hip findings in asymptomatic participants: a prospective, blinded study. Am J Sports Med 2012;40(12):2720–4. http://dx.doi.org/10.1177/0363546512462124.
39. Schmitz MR, Campbell SE, Fajardo RS, et al. Identification of acetabular labral pathological changes in asymptomatic volunteers using optimized, noncontrast 1.5-T magnetic resonance imaging. Am J Sports Med 2012;40(6):1337–41. http://dx.doi.org/10.1177/0363546512439991.
40. Byrd JW. Patient selection and physical examination. In: Byrd JW, editor. Operative hip arthroscopy. 3rd edition. New York: Springer; 2013. p. 7–33. http://dx.doi.org/10.1007/978-1-4419-7925-4.
41. Martin HD. Clinical examination and imaging of the hip. In: Byrd JT, Guanche CA, editors. AANA advanced arthroscopy: the hip. Philadelphia: Elsevier; 2010. p. 3–30.
42. Ochoa LM, Dawson L, Patzkowski JC, et al. Radiographic prevalence of femoroacetabular impingement in a young population with hip complaints is high. Clin Orthop Relat Res 2010;468(10):2710–4. http://dx.doi.org/10.1007/s11999-010-1233-8.
43. Clohisy JC, Carlisle JC, Beaulé PE, et al. A systematic approach to the plain radiographic evaluation of the young adult hip. J Bone Joint Surg Am 2008; 90(Suppl 4):47–66. http://dx.doi.org/10.2106/JBJS.H.00756.

44. Tannast M, Siebenrock KA, Anderson SE. Femoroacetabular impingement: radiographic diagnosis–what the radiologist should know. AJR Am J Roentgenol 2007;188(6):1540–52. http://dx.doi.org/10.2214/AJR.06.0921.

45. Chang CY, Huang AJ. MR imaging of normal hip anatomy. Magn Reson Imaging Clin N Am 2013;21(1):1–19. http://dx.doi.org/10.1016/j.mric.2012.08.006.

46. Byrd JW. Diagnostic accuracy of clinical assessment, magnetic resonance imaging, magnetic resonance arthrography, and intra-articular injection in hip arthroscopy patients. Am J Sports Med 2004;32(7):1668–74. http://dx.doi.org/10.1177/0363546504266480.

47. Byrd JW. Cam-type femoroacetabular impingement. In: Thomas Byrd JW, Guanche CA, editors. AANA advanced arthroscopy: the hip. Philadelphia: Elsevier; 2010. p. 65–78.

48. Byrd JW. Femoroacetabular impingement in athletes: current concepts. Am J Sports Med 2013;42:737–51. http://dx.doi.org/10.1177/0363546513499136.

49. Heyworth BE, Dolan MM, Nguyen JT, et al. Preoperative three-dimensional CT predicts intraoperative findings in hip arthroscopy. Clin Orthop Relat Res 2012;470(7):1950–7. http://dx.doi.org/10.1007/s11999-012-2331-6.

50. Byrd JW, Potts EA, Allison RK, et al. Ultrasound-guided hip injections: a comparative study with fluoroscopy-guided injections. Arthroscopy 2014;30(1):42–6. http://dx.doi.org/10.1016/j.arthro.2013.09.083.

51. Nepple JJ, Byrd JW, Siebenrock KA, et al. Overview of treatment options, clinical results, and controversies in the management of femoroacetabular impingement. J Am Acad Orthop Surg 2013;21(Suppl 1):S53–8. http://dx.doi.org/10.5435/JAAOS-21-07-S53.

52. Quinn A. Hip and groin pain: physiotherapy and rehabilitation issues. Open Sports Med J 2010;4:93–107.

53. Birmingham PM, Kelly BT, Jacobs R, et al. The effect of dynamic femoroacetabular impingement on pubic symphysis motion: a cadaveric study. Am J Sports Med 2012;40(5):1113–8. http://dx.doi.org/10.1177/0363546512437723.

54. Colvin AC, Harrast J, Harner C. Trends in hip arthroscopy. J Bone Joint Surg Am 2012;94(4):e23. http://dx.doi.org/10.2106/JBJS.J.01886.

55. Montgomery SR, Ngo SS, Hobson T, et al. Trends and demographics in hip arthroscopy in the United States. Arthroscopy 2013;29(4):661–5. http://dx.doi.org/10.1016/j.arthro.2012.11.005.

56. Jacoby L, Yi-Meng Y, Kocher MS. Hip problems and arthroscopy: adolescent hip as it relates to sports. Clin Sports Med 2011;30(2):435–51. http://dx.doi.org/10.1016/j.csm.2011.01.003.

57. Lubowitz JH, Poehling GG. Hip arthroscopy: an emerging gold standard. Arthroscopy 2006;22(12):1257–9. http://dx.doi.org/10.1016/j.arthro.2006.10.002.

58. Clarke MT, Arora A, Villar RN. Hip arthroscopy: complications in 1054 cases. Clin Orthop Relat Res 2003;(406):84–8. http://dx.doi.org/10.1097/01.blo.0000043048.84315.af.

59. Bogunovic L, Gottlieb M, Pashos G, et al. Why do hip arthroscopy procedures fail? Clin Orthop Relat Res 2013;471:2523–9. http://dx.doi.org/10.1007/s11999-013-3015-6.

60. Bedi A, Zbeda RM, Bueno VF, et al. The incidence of heterotopic ossification after hip arthroscopy. Am J Sports Med 2012;40(4):854–63. http://dx.doi.org/10.1177/0363546511434285.

61. Hoppe DJ, de Sa D, Simunovic N, et al. The learning curve for hip arthroscopy: a systematic review. Arthroscopy 2014;30(3):389–97. http://dx.doi.org/10.1016/j.arthro.2013.11.012.

62. Byrd JW. Hip arthroscopy utilizing the supine position. Arthroscopy 1994;10(3): 275–80. Available at: http://www.ncbi.nlm.nih.gov/pubmed/8777012. Accessed December 16, 2013.

63. Keene GS, Villar RN. Arthroscopic anatomy of the hip: an in vivo study. Arthroscopy 1994;10(4):392–9. Available at: http://www.ncbi.nlm.nih.gov/pubmed/7945634.

64. McCarthy JC, Lee JA. History of hip arthroscopy: challenges and opportunities. Clin Sports Med 2011;30(2):217–24. http://dx.doi.org/10.1016/j.csm.2010.12.001.

65. Byrd JW. Hip arthroscopy. J Am Acad Orthop Surg 2006;14(7):433–44. Available at: http://www.ncbi.nlm.nih.gov/pubmed/22989716.

66. Kelly BT, Weiland DE, Schenker ML, et al. Arthroscopic labral repair in the hip: surgical technique and review of the literature. Arthroscopy 2005;21(12): 1496–504. http://dx.doi.org/10.1016/j.arthro.2005.08.013.

67. Philippon MJ, Stubbs AJ, Schenker ML, et al. Arthroscopic management of femoroacetabular impingement: osteoplasty technique and literature review. Am J Sports Med 2007;35(9):1571–80. http://dx.doi.org/10.1177/0363546507300258.

68. Bond JL, Knutson ZA, Ebert A, et al. The 23-point arthroscopic examination of the hip: basic setup, portal placement, and surgical technique. Arthroscopy 2009;25(4):416–29. http://dx.doi.org/10.1016/j.arthro.2008.08.021.

69. Byrd JW, Pappas JN, Pedley MJ. Hip arthroscopy: an anatomic study of portal placement and relationship to the extra-articular structures. Arthroscopy 1995; 11(4):418–23. Available at: http://www.ncbi.nlm.nih.gov/pubmed/7575873.

70. Robertson WJ, Kelly BT. The safe zone for hip arthroscopy: a cadaveric assessment of central, peripheral, and lateral compartment portal placement. Arthroscopy 2008;24(9):1019–26. http://dx.doi.org/10.1016/j.arthro.2008.05.008.

71. Philippon MJ, Weiss DR, Kuppersmith DA, et al. Arthroscopic labral repair and treatment of femoroacetabular impingement in professional hockey players. Am J Sports Med 2010;38(1):99–104. http://dx.doi.org/10.1177/0363546509346393.

72. Byrd JW. Labral lesions: an elusive source of hip pain case reports and literature review. Arthroscopy 1996;12(5):603–12. Available at: http://www.ncbi.nlm.nih.gov/pubmed/8902136. Accessed June 12, 2013.

73. Tibor LM, Leunig M. Labral resection or preservation during FAI treatment? A systematic review. HSS J 2012;8(3):225–9. http://dx.doi.org/10.1007/s11420-012-9294-8.

74. Larson CM, Giveans MR, Stone RM. Arthroscopic debridement versus refixation of the acetabular labrum associated with femoroacetabular impingement: mean 3.5-year follow-up. Am J Sports Med 2012;40(5):1015–21. http://dx.doi.org/10.1177/0363546511434578.

75. Espinosa N, Rothenfluh DA, Beck M, et al. Treatment of femoro-acetabular impingement: preliminary results of labral refixation. J Bone Joint Surg Am 2006;88(5):925–35. http://dx.doi.org/10.2106/JBJS.E.00290.

76. Harris JD, Erickson BJ, Bush-Joseph CA, et al. Treatment of femoroacetabular impingement: a systematic review. Curr Rev Musculoskelet Med 2013;6(3): 207–18. http://dx.doi.org/10.1007/s12178-013-9172-0.

77. Heyworth BE, Shindle MK, Voos JE, et al. Radiologic and intraoperative findings in revision hip arthroscopy. Arthroscopy 2007;23(12):1295–302. http://dx.doi.org/10.1016/j.arthro.2007.09.015.

78. Philippon MJ, Schenker ML, Briggs KK, et al. Revision hip arthroscopy. Am J Sports Med 2007;35(11):1918–21. http://dx.doi.org/10.1177/0363546507305097.

79. Tannast M, Goricki D, Beck M, et al. Hip damage occurs at the zone of femoroacetabular impingement. Clin Orthop Relat Res 2008;466(2):273–80. http://dx.doi.org/10.1007/s11999-007-0061-y.

80. McDonald JE, Herzog MM, Philippon MJ. Return to play after hip arthroscopy with microfracture in elite athletes. Arthroscopy 2013;29(2):330–5. http://dx. doi.org/10.1016/j.arthro.2012.08.028.
81. Karthikeyan S, Roberts S, Griffin D. Microfracture for acetabular chondral defects in patients with femoroacetabular impingement: results at second-look arthroscopic surgery. Am J Sports Med 2012;40(12):2725–30. http://dx.doi. org/10.1177/0363546512465400.
82. Jordan MA, Van Thiel GS, Chahal J, et al. Operative treatment of chondral defects in the hip joint: a systematic review. Curr Rev Musculoskelet Med 2012; 5(3):244–53. http://dx.doi.org/10.1007/s12178-012-9134-y.
83. Byrd JW. Femoroacetabular impingement in athletes, part 1: cause and assessment. Sports Health 2010;2(4):321–33. http://dx.doi.org/10.1177/1941738110368392.
84. Ross JR, Bedi A, Stone RM, et al. Intraoperative fluoroscopic imaging to treat cam deformities: correlation with 3-dimensional computed tomography. Am J Sports Med 2014;42(6):1370–6. http://dx.doi.org/10.1177/0363546514529515.
85. Philippon MJ, Souza BG. Femoroacetabular impingement: pincer. In: Byrd JW, Guanche CA, editors. AANA advanced arthroscopy: the hip. Philadelphia: Elsevier; 2010. p. 79–89.
86. Byrd JW. Hip arthroscopy in the athlete. Oper Tech Sports Med 2012;20(4): 310–9. http://dx.doi.org/10.1053/j.otsm.2012.08.003.
87. Leunig M, Beaulé PE, Ganz R. The concept of femoroacetabular impingement: current status and future perspectives. Clin Orthop Relat Res 2009;467(3): 616–22. http://dx.doi.org/10.1007/s11999-008-0646-0.
88. Byrd JW, Jones KS. Arthroscopic femoroplasty in the management of cam-type femoroacetabular impingement. Clin Orthop Relat Res 2009;467(3):739–46. http://dx.doi.org/10.1007/s11999-008-0659-8.

Management of Chronic Lateral Ankle Instability in Military Service Members

Justin D. Orr, MD[a,b,]*, Justin Robbins, MD[c],
Brian R. Waterman, MD[a,b]

KEYWORDS

- Ankle instability • Lateral instability • Ankle sprain • Chronic • Military • Treatment

KEY POINTS

- Chronic lateral ankle instability is a condition frequently encountered by orthopedic surgeons treating highly active patient populations, particularly military service members.
- Providers treating military service members must have a high index of suspicion for this condition when signs and symptoms of functional or mechanical instability exist.
- Stress testing and ankle magnetic resonance imaging, although not definitive in sensitivity for detecting instability or other concomitant injuries, should be considered during the treatment decision-making process.
- Appropriate nonoperative treatment should be attempted initially; however, when nonoperative treatment fails, surgical management is warranted to prevent untoward long-term sequelae.
- Proper surgical treatment and subsequent postoperative management are at the discretion of the individual surgeon but must account for the concomitant diseases frequently associated with chronic lateral ankle instability.
- Low recurrence of lateral instability can be achieved even in high-demand military patient populations with a focused treatment plan.

INTRODUCTION AND EPIDEMIOLOGY

Acute lateral, or inversion, ankle sprains are among the most common musculoskeletal injuries encountered in military patients. Within the civilian population, daily estimates of acute and subacute ankle sprains range from 5000 per day in the United Kingdom to as high as 23,000 to 30,000 in other societies such as the United States.[1–6] Overall, ankle sprains account for an estimated 10% to 40% of civilian athletic injuries annually and can result in significant time lost to injury.[5,7–10] The mainstay of

[a] William Beaumont Army Medical Center, 5005 N. Piedras Street, El Paso, TX 79920, USA;
[b] Department of Orthopaedic Surgery, Texas Tech University Health Sciences Center, El Paso, Texas; [c] Madigan Army Medical Center, 9040 Jackson Avenue, Tacoma, WA 98431, USA
* Corresponding author.
E-mail address: Justin.d.orr.mil@mail.mil

Clin Sports Med 33 (2014) 675–692
http://dx.doi.org/10.1016/j.csm.2014.06.011
0278-5919/14/$ – see front matter Published by Elsevier Inc.
sportsmed.theclinics.com

management for acute inversion ankle sprains remains nonoperative treatment, typically with early immobilization and functional rehabilitation, focusing on achievement of full range of motion, peroneal tendon strengthening and proprioception, and gradual progression of weight bearing as tolerated.[4,10,11] A rich body of evidence exists showing no significant improvement in long-term functional outcomes when high-grade acute lateral ankle sprains are initially managed operatively compared with nonoperatively with early functional rehabilitation.[12-15] Despite appropriate nonoperative management after acute inversion ankle sprains, 10% to 30% of individuals have recurrences of instability and progress to chronic symptomatic lateral ankle instability.[2,5,6,16-18] Repeated inversion ankle sprains can propagate osteochondral lesions of the talus (OCLT),[18,19] chronic peroneal tendinopathy,[4,20-22] peroneal neuropathy,[23] varus malalignment, and risk for early tibiotalar osteoarthritis.[4,21,22] Given the increased rate of ankle sprains in athletic populations, coupled with high recurrence rates and the potential for disabling long-term sequelae, management of chronic lateral ankle instability in high-demand military and populations poses significant challenges for orthopedic surgeons.

The US military armed forces represent a diverse, physically active population, with generally high occupational demands. Service members participate in organized physical fitness training programs and must meet the standards of the physical fitness tests of their individual services as well as height and weight requirements semiannually.[24] The active duty service population is not unlike athletic populations in civilian cohorts. Military personnel consistently train on and are deployed to regions with a multitude of uneven surfaces, carrying combat loads often exceeding 45 kg (100 lb). They are at increased risk for inversion ankle sprains and subsequent chronic lateral ankle instability. Waterman and colleagues[25] reported on the incidence of ankle sprains in cadets at the US Military Academy (USMA) in West Point, New York, and noted an overall incidence rate of 58.4 sprains per 1000 person-years, regardless of participation in intercollegiate versus mandatory intramural athletics. These results suggest that inversion ankle sprains, the precipitant of chronic lateral ankle instability, may be more common in military than civilian populations. Orr and colleagues[24] reported on the increased incidence of OCLTs among US military personnel, with significant progressive increases in incidence noted throughout the years of overseas conflict from 2002 to 2008. The investigators cited the likely relationship between increasing ankle instability and its role in causing more OCLTs. The lead author of this review performed approximately 75 primary and revision lateral ligamentous reconstructions annually between 2009 and 2013 at a large tertiary care military medical treatment facility servicing a high volume of active duty military personnel.

In this review, the anatomy, risk factors, and clinical presentation associated with chronic lateral ankle instability are discussed, as well as preferred nonoperative and operative treatment strategies in military populations. The nuances of early diagnosis and management of acute ankle sprains are beyond the scope of this review. We have focused specifically on management of chronic instability within the military population. These same principles are valid when considering treatment of this condition in other physically active patient populations, whose activity demands are through sports or high-demand occupational activities.

ANATOMY AND CAUSE

The lateral ligamentous complex can best be thought of as a capsuloligamentous complex, because the anterolateral joint capsule contributes to the ligamentous stability of the lateral ankle. The ligamentous complex consists of 3 ligaments: anterior talofibular ligament (ATFL), calcaneofibular ligament (CFL), and posterior talofibular ligament (PTFL). The ATFL is contiguous with the anterolateral joint capsule, representing a discrete intracapsular thickening, originating on the anteroinferior border of the lateral malleolus and inserting on the lateral talar neck.[26,27] Just posteriorly adjacent to the ATFL origin, the CFL originates on the distal fibula. It is an extracapsular structure, coursing obliquely to its insertion on the lateral calcaneal tubercle, traversing the tibiotalar and subtalar joints.[26,27] Biomechanically, the thicker CFL is stronger than the ATFL.[26] The largest and strongest of the 3 ligaments, the PTFL is rarely injured during typical inversion ankle sprains.[6,26]

Lateral ankle stability requires both dynamic and static constraints. Dynamic stability is provided most directly from the strength of the peroneal tendons and through involuntary proprioceptive feedback.[28,29] Static stability is provided by osseous anatomy as well as ligamentous, retinacular, and capsular constraints. The primary static ligamentous stabilizers are the ATFL and CFL.[26,29–31] The ATFL serves as the primary constraint to anterior talar translation and talar inversion during plantarflexion.[32,33] Similarly, the CFL serves as the primary constraint to talar inversion in neutral and dorsiflexion.[32,33] The ATFL is injured more commonly in inversion ankle sprains than the CFL.[31,34–36] Evidence by Broström[35] showed intraoperative ATFL tears in all patients with chronic lateral ankle instability; however, there were no isolated CFL tears. It is likely given the role of ATFL as the primary static ligamentous constraint to talar inversion in plantarflexion that it is more prone to injury during inversion ankle sprains. This concept has been reproduced biomechanically, because inversion stress with progressive plantarflexion produces significantly more strain on the ATFL compared with the CFL.[37] Subsequently, many investigators historically address only the ATFL during primary lateral ligamentous reconstruction.[21,35]

Most inversion lateral ankle sprains, whether acute or recurrent, occur after axial loading on an externally rotated leg with excessive inversion of the hindfoot. The ankle may be in any position, but most commonly is plantarflexed. This situation places maximum stress on the lateral ligamentous complex, particularly the weaker ATFL. The ATFL is 3 times more likely than the CFL to be injured in cases of acute or chronic ankle instability.[27,38]

RISK FACTORS FOR CHRONIC LATERAL ANKLE INSTABILITY

Waterman and colleagues[39,40] identified several nonmodifiable and modifiable risk factors for development of lateral ankle instability. Specifically, nonmodifiable risk factors noted by these investigators included gender, age, and previous ankle sprain. In addition, increased body mass index (BMI) and presence of hindfoot or midfoot malalignment conditions as well as poor neuromuscular postural control (proprioception) can predispose one to chronic lateral ankle instability.

Gender does seem to play a role in the development of chronic lateral ankle instability. A recent epidemiologic study by Waterman and colleagues[25] found that in cadets at USMA, the adjusted incidence rate ratio for ankle sprains in female cadets was 1.83 compared with matched male cadets. As well, a recent prospective randomized controlled trial by Frey and colleagues[41] compared the incidence of lateral ankle instability in 957 high-school volleyball players who wore prophylactic rigid, semirigid, and nonrigid ankle braces with controls without braces. Although the study did not find significant benefit from use of ankle bracing in athletes with a history of lateral ankle instability, it did note a significantly increased incidence of inversion ankle sprains in female athletes wearing nonrigid braces compared with men wearing the same type of brace. This finding may represent a natural tendency toward increased ligamentous laxity in women compared with men, as has been described with anterior cruciate ligament laxity.[42,43] Female service members account for 13.5% of all US Army forces.[44] Because female service members are expected to perform the same rigorous physical training as male service members, possible increased ligamentous laxity and resultant increased ankle instability may contribute to a higher incidence of chronic lateral ankle instability in female service members. Age also seems critical to the development of chronic lateral ankle instability. Younger age, as would be expected in military personnel, is associated with increased risk of ankle sprain and subsequent chronic lateral ankle instability. A recent population-based study within an active duty service member population[45] reported the highest incidence rates for ankle sprain (the forerunner of chronic lateral ankle instability) in military populations younger than 20 years, regardless of gender.

In addition, increased BMI has been shown to increase the likelihood of lateral ankle instability. Epidemiologic data have shown significantly higher incidences of ankle sprains in patients with increased BMI, because increased body weight imparts more exertional forces across the lateral ankle during axial loading activities.[25,46] Although most active duty service members are physically fit secondary to stringent height-related BMI restrictions, military personnel are expected to carry heavy combat loads, often exceeding 45 kg (100 lb), over uneven terrains.

Previous ankle sprains are sometimes harbingers of later chronic lateral ankle instability.[2,5,6,16,17,28,47,48] Other investigators have reported that after even a single inversion ankle sprain, there exists altered ankle proprioception, decreased peroneal tendon strength and function, and accumulation of inflammatory scar tissue in the injured capsuloligamentous complex.[4,28,48–50] As well, previous investigators[28,48,49] have reported that reduced peroneal tendon strength can result in reduced proprioception and resultant lateral ankle instability. Other risk factors for development of chronic lateral ankle instability include anatomic malalignment conditions and impaired proprioception. Specifically, hindfoot varus, midfoot cavus, or combined cavovarus deformities predispose patients to lateral ankle instability by abnormally altering normal hindfoot alignment and placing untoward stress on the lateral ligamentous complex and peroneal tendons.[51,52] Similarly, impaired proprioception, especially when combined with a previous ankle sprain, has been shown to increase risk of chronic lateral ankle instability.[28,48,50,53–57]

CLINICAL PRESENTATION

Assessment of military service members with suspected chronic lateral ankle instability should include a complete patient history to assess the service member's chief complaint, previous mechanisms and degrees of injuries, previous nonoperative and operative treatments, and current levels of activity and limitations. Although presentations of acute ankle inversion injuries are often more obvious to the examiner, the clinical presentation of persistent, chronic lateral ankle instability may be more insidious and subtle. Military patients on active duty often articulate feelings of giving way or rolling on both flat and uneven surfaces. Regarding daily activities, a service member will use terms such as loose, weak, and unsteady to describe their ankle. Service members may describe a sense of apprehension while walking on uneven surfaces. Commonly, pain is not a persistent complaint and more commonly accompanies new ankle sprains. If ankle pain is persistent, then, other concomitant injuries should be suspected, such as anterior ankle soft tissue or osseous impingement; ankle synovitis; OCLT(s); syndesmotic injury; associated fractures about the ankle, hindfoot, and midfoot; peroneal tendinopathy(s); intra-articular loose body(s); peripheral neuropathy (ie, peroneal nerve and associated branches); or early-onset degenerative joint disease. In our opinion, one of the most crucial series of questions that should be asked of all military patients is: (1) "Does it seem that you have a sharp pain, followed by rolling the ankle?" and (2) "Does it seem that you roll the ankle and have pain afterward?" This is an important factor during the initial clinical evaluation, because pain that causes instability could be a sign of mechanical factors such as loose body(s), OCLT(s) (**Fig. 1**), anterior impingement, or anterior synovitis, which can be mitigated without formal lateral ligamentous reconstruction.

PHYSICAL EXAMINATION

All patients with suspected chronic lateral ankle instability should undergo a thorough examination of both lower extremities. Typically, we assess standing alignment first. Particular attention is given to the presence of hindfoot varus, midfoot cavus, or combined cavovarus deformities (**Fig. 2**), because these conditions must be addressed at the time of any successful lateral ligamentous reconstruction.[51,52] Next, a thorough neurovascular examination should be performed. Special attention is given to any peroneal nerve dysfunction, because repeated lateral ankle sprains place untoward tensile stress on the nerve fibers and can propagate peroneal neuropathy.[23] Palpation about the ankle is important as well, and focus should be given to palpation of the anterior ankle joint to identify possible anterior synovitis or joint effusion. In addition, the presence of a sulcus sign just anterior to the lateral malleolus is an indicator of lack of ATFL continuity. Initial assessment should include evaluation of bilateral ankle and subtalar joint ranges of motion with notation of any pain or crepitus during range of motion. During examination, if there is any indication of generalized ligamentous laxity, then a complete evaluation for joint hypermobility must be conducted in accordance with the Beighton scoring system,[58] because generalized ligamentous laxity can alter the treatment decision-making process.

A full motor strength examination should be performed, but special attention is given to the peroneal tendon examination. A dedicated peroneal tendon examination should

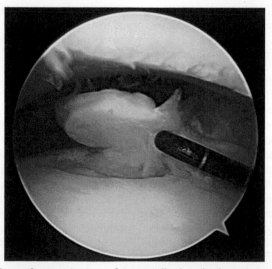

Fig. 1. Intraoperative arthroscopic view of a partially detached centrolateral osteochondral lesion of the talus.

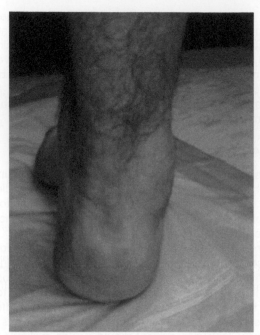

Fig. 2. Clinical presentation of patient with cavovarus deformity, contributing to chronic lateral ankle instability.

be performed to determine the possibility of peroneal tendinopathy or instability. Chronic lateral ankle instability may lead to primary or secondary chronic peroneal tendinopathy.[4,20–22,59] The strength of the peroneus brevis muscle, the primary hindfoot everter, is determined by evaluating resisted ankle plantarflexion with simultaneous hindfoot eversion. Direct palpation over the peroneal tendons during resisted plantarflexion and eversion can elicit isolated peroneal tendon pain or fullness (**Fig. 3**), suggestive of tenosynovitis or tendon tears (ie, longitudinal split tears). The examiner must evaluate for possible peroneal instability. Although peroneal tendon instability is rare, if present, it must be addressed just as with any other peroneal tendon condition at the time of lateral ligamentous reconstruction.[20,60]

STRESS TESTING

Routine use of dynamic, fluoroscopic-assisted stress testing is controversial, and most investigators agree that stress test results should not be a dominant factor in determining surgical candidacy.[4,6,22,61] We advocate anterior drawer and talar tilt fluoroscopic stress testing in every patient with suspected chronic lateral ankle instability for treatment decision making. Traditionally, the anterior drawer stress test is performed in plantarflexion, with attempted anterior translation of the talus in relation to the tibia. Because the ATFL is the primary restraint to anterior talar translation,[32,33] the anterior drawer stress test most reliably evaluates integrity of the ATFL. The talar tilt stress test is performed in dorsiflexion, with attempted inversion or varus tilting of the talus within the mortise. Because the CFL is the primary restraint to talar inversion in dorsiflexion,[32,33] this examination most reliably evaluates the integrity of the CFL. However, the ATFL is the primary restraint to talar inversion in ankle plantarflexion.[32,33] Thus, a talar tilt stress test performed in plantarflexion evaluates integrity of the ATFL

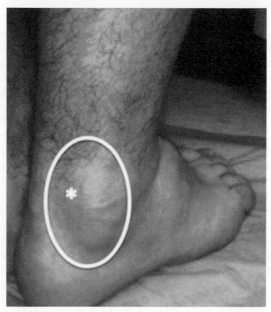

Fig. 3. Clinical presentation of patient with chronic lateral ankle instability and associated peroneal fullness (*asterisk*).

as well. For this reason, the ability to identify specific ligamentous disease based on stress testing results is questionable.[62] Furthermore, there is an unknown contribution from the subtalar joint, especially in cases with concomitant subtalar instability, to the talar tilt stress test.[61] We believe that an anterior drawer 3 to 5 mm greater than the uninjured side is suspicious for abnormality.[4,5,22,62] Similarly, we believe that a talar tilt in both dorsiflexion and plantarflexion of 5° greater than the uninjured side is suspicious for ligamentous abnormality.[4,5,22,62]

FUNCTIONAL VERSUS MECHANICAL INSTABILITY

Functional instability implies loss of voluntary control to maintain lateral ankle stability on unforgiving surfaces that military populations are frequently exposed to (ie, uneven terrain, rocks, and gravel).[63] It has been postulated that functional instability is secondary to loss of normal proprioception and neuromuscular control.[22,63,64] Service members with functional instability describe a feeling of giving way or rolling on uneven surfaces. In our military patient populations, to determine if functional instability exists, we routinely ask service members the following questions: (1) "Do you feel like your ankle gives way on uneven surfaces?" and (2) "Do you frequently roll your ankle during training and on uneven surfaces?" Conversely, mechanical instability implies loss of normal anatomic constraint to lateral ankle stability. It is usually identifiable on physical examination in the form of abnormal stress testing or generalized laxity. Several investigators[38,65] agree that the 2 forms of instability rarely occur in isolation. Instead, most chronic lateral ankle instability is a combination of functional and mechanical instability, with increased lateral ligamentous laxity necessarily accompanied by impaired proprioception.[38,65–67] In our experience, it is a service member's functional instability that prompts an orthopedic surgical evaluation. In the military population, it is the presence of functional instability and not isolated, asymptomatic mechanical instability that warrants intervention.

RADIOGRAPHY

Initial radiographic evaluation of all service members with suspected chronic lateral ankle instability begins with weight-bearing ankle radiographs to assess for missed ankle and hindfoot fractures, early degenerative changes, and other associated injuries. As discussed earlier, we routinely evaluate fluoroscopic-assisted stress testing. We universally obtain magnetic resonance imaging (MRI) of the ankle in all cases of confirmed chronic lateral ankle instability. Some investigators do not encourage routine ankle MRI in patients with chronic lateral ankle instability.[4-6] O'Neill and colleagues[68] reported that ankle MRI had a sensitivity of only 63% for detection of OCLTs, loose bodies, and peroneal tendon tears in patients with lateral ankle instability. Other investigators have reported higher sensitivity at detecting OCLTs and peroneal tendon tears.[69] The overall level of evidence is insufficient to recommend in favor of or against routine use of ankle MRI. We prefer to obtain MRI, especially in operative candidates, to help determine the need for concomitant ankle arthroscopy, peroneal tendon exploration, or larger cartilage restorative surgery secondary to OCLT(s) (**Fig. 4**A). Ankle MRI can best detect the presence of an abnormal ATFL on axial T2-weighted sequences (see **Fig. 4**B). Similarly, ankle MRI can best detect the presence of an abnormal CFL on coronal T2-weighted sequences (see **Fig. 4**C). Suspicion of ATFL or CFL abnormalities based solely on MRI does not indicate surgical management of lateral ligamentous instability but simply should be used (just as with stress testing results) during treatment decision making. Ankle MRI can elucidate the presence of anterolateral ankle synovitis (see **Fig. 4**B) or the presence of peroneal tendon disease (see **Fig. 4**D), both of which affect operative planning.

NONOPERATIVE MANAGEMENT

Early functional rehabilitation should be the initial treatment of first-time lateral ankle sprains. There is no advantage with early operative management of acute ankle sprains compared with nonoperative management incorporating initial immobilization, RICE (rest, ice, compression, and elevation) therapy, early range of motion and physical therapy, and progression of weight bearing as tolerated.[12-15,70]

In military patient populations, we prefer an initial 2-month to 3-month course of structured physical therapy before consideration of operative management. Although other investigators have recommended shorter periods of nonoperative management,[4-6,22] we concur with previous investigators who have recommended at least 2 to 3 months of attempted nonoperative treatment.[17,21,71] Patients who present with chronic lateral ankle instability, particularly functional or combined functional and mechanical instability, are immediately started on a physical therapy program that incorporates range of motion, peroneal tendon strengthening, and proprioceptive exercises.[48,54,72] Nonoperative treatment of functional instability focuses on improvement in balance and proprioception. To this end, many physical therapists incorporate the use of a biomechanical ankle platform system (BAPS) board (**Fig. 5**).[54,63,72,73] Improvement in mechanical instability is directed toward motor strengthening, particularly the peroneal tendons, through a directed course of active and passive strengthening regimens in conjunction with proprioceptive therapy.[28,48,49] In general, the athletic patient or military service member with purely functional instability is more likely to benefit from nonoperative management compared with those with combined functional and mechanical instability.[74]

In addition, the investigators routinely recommend use of semirigid ankle stabilizers (braces) in military service members undergoing a 2-month to 3-month nonoperative treatment program. The efficacy of semirigid ankle braces has been questioned, with

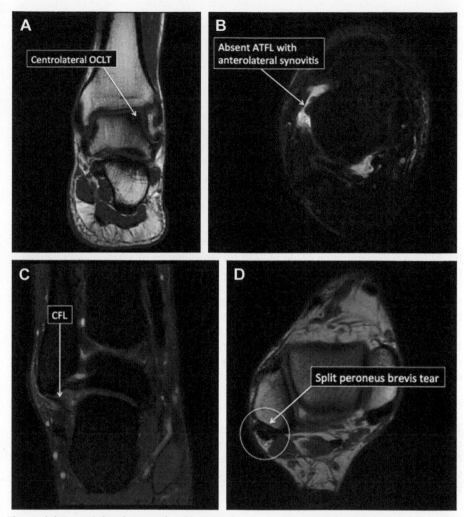

Fig. 4. (*A*) T1-weighted coronal ankle MRI showing centrolateral osteochondral lesion of the talus. (*B*) T2-weighted axial ankle MRI showing suspected chronic ATFL injury with associated anterolateral synovitis. (*C*) T2-weighted coronal ankle MRI showing normal- appearing CFL. (*D*) T1-weighted axial ankle MRI showing suspected longitudinal split tear of the peroneus brevis tendon.

some investigators noting reduction in episodes of instability[11,73,75] and other investigators[41] finding no benefit in athletes with diagnosed chronic lateral ankle instability. Regardless, we believe that semirigid ankle braces can provide valuable protection for military personnel, frequently exposed to unforgiving, uneven terrains during physical and military training, as they undergo therapy to restore peroneal tendon strength and proprioception. A variety of commercially available semirigid ankle braces exist that include strap (**Fig. 6**A; DJO Global Aircast, Vista, CA) or lace-up (see **Fig. 6**B; DJO Global Procare, Vista, CA) designs. All incorporate some type of low-profile anatomically molded semirigid medial and lateral plastic supports. These ankle braces may be difficult to comfortably fit into a standard military working boot. Therefore, we find that

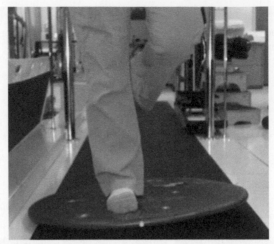

Fig. 5. Clinical demonstration of use of BAPS for rehabilitation of a patient with functional chronic lateral ankle instability.

most service members refrain from use of the semirigid ankle brace during military boot wear and prefer to use the braces only with athletic shoe wear. The overall level of evidence is insufficient to recommend in favor of or against routine use of ankle bracing in these patients. Military service members undergoing nonoperative management for chronic lateral ankle instability are also placed on stringent work-related activity limitations.

OPERATIVE MANAGEMENT

The primary indication for operative management of chronic lateral ankle instability is continued instability after an appropriate course of comprehensive nonoperative management. Appropriate nonoperative management implies that the service member completed a 2-month to 3-month course of therapy and was consistently compliant with therapy and activity restrictions throughout the treatment course. In 2006,

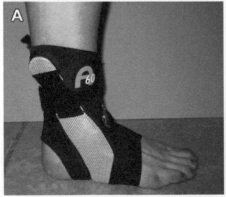
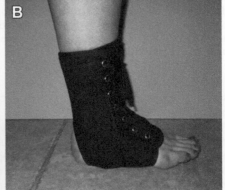

Fig. 6. (*A*) Clinical photograph showing semirigid strap design ankle brace. (*B*) Clinical photograph showing semirigid lace-up design ankle brace. (*Courtesy of* DJO Global Aircast, Vista, CA; with permission.)

DiGiovanni and Brodsky[4] provided a comprehensive current concepts review of each of the most relevant lateral ligamentous reconstructive procedures and the most popular modifications of each procedure. A complete discussion of these operative procedures is outside the context and scope of this review. Therefore, we have focused on our operative treatment preferences for military personnel with chronic lateral ankle instability, cognizant that no singular, best operative technique exists. Furthermore, the nuances of revision lateral ligament reconstruction when primary reconstruction has failed are outside the context of this review.

Operative reconstruction techniques can be classified as anatomic, nonanatomic, or anatomic tenodesis reconstructions.[4,22] The foundation of anatomic reconstruction techniques is the Broström repair, described in 1966.[35] Regardless of technique, the goal of all anatomic reconstructions is to restore lateral ligamentous integrity and maintain ankle and subtalar joint kinematics. Numerous studies have reported good to excellent outcomes in more than 85% of patients using a variety of anatomic lateral ligamentous repairs for treatment of chronic lateral ankle instability.[17,21,35,71,76–83] Common to all nonanatomic reconstructions is transosseous rerouting and tenodesis of local tendon autografts (ie, peroneus brevis tendon) to restore lateral ankle stability. These techniques have consistently had poor long-term outcomes secondary to altered ankle and subtalar joint kinetics.[4,22,84,85] Anatomic tenodesis reconstructions are numerous and involve augmentation of anatomic reconstructions by splitting the peroneus brevis tendon and tenodesing the tensioned tendon through transosseous tunnels or directly to the primary anatomic repair itself. Although overtightening is possible with this technique, clinical results have been favorable and indicate that this augmentation may preserve normal ankle and subtalar joint kinematics with the added benefit of enhanced repair strength.[71,86,87]

Role of Ankle Arthroscopy

The overall level of evidence is insufficient to recommend in favor of or against routine ankle arthroscopy in all primary lateral ankle ligamentous reconstructions.[4,22] However, several investigators[18,19,88,89] support routine ankle arthroscopy for these patients, citing high incidences of intra-articular disease and OCLTs in as many as 25% of patients. However, not all investigators routinely obtain preoperative ankle MRI before lateral ligamentous reconstruction as we do. The ability of ankle MRI to successfully identify intra-articular disease such as loose bodies and OCLTs has yielded mixed results.[68,69] The advantages of not performing arthroscopy before lateral ligamentous reconstruction are easier patient positioning and a more clearly defined soft tissue envelope during the open procedure. We use the following algorithm in our military population undergoing lateral ankle ligamentous reconstructions:

1. All patients undergo preoperative ankle MRI
2. If ankle MRI shows intra-articular pathology → ankle arthroscopy
3. If ankle MRI is inconclusive or negative for intra-articular pathology(s), and intra-articular ankle pain is a predominant presenting symptom → ankle arthroscopy
4. If ankle MRI is inconclusive or negative for intra-articular pathology(s), and intra-articular ankle pain is not a predominant presenting symptom → no ankle arthroscopy

Our Preferred Treatment of Primary Lateral Ligamentous Reconstruction

In military service members who have failed appropriate nonoperative treatment of chronic lateral ankle instability, we prefer anatomic reconstruction. Specifically, we routinely perform a modified Broström technique,[35,78] using a lateral capsuloliga-mentous imbrication similar to Karlsson and colleagues' description.[76,77] The repair is secured with suture anchors and reinforced with a local distal fibular periosteal flap similar to previous investigators' descriptions.[81,82,90] In rare cases when the local soft tissues are less than optimal, we typically enhance the reconstruction with local split peroneus brevis tendon, as described by previous investigators.[86,87]

The procedure is typically performed under general anesthetic with a thigh or calf tourniquet. If diagnostic arthroscopy is performed before ligament reconstruction, the patient is placed in a semilateral position on a beanbag to best facilitate both procedures. If no arthroscopy is performed, the patient is placed in a direct lateral position on a beanbag. With regard to the lateral ligament reconstruction, a curvilinear incision is made over the lateral ankle. We prefer the lateral curvilinear approach because of its versatility to allow for proximal and distal extension. We first identify and isolate the inferior extensor retinaculum (IER) for later augmentation (**Fig. 7**A). It is critical to meticulously identify and dissect the IER from the underlying tissues to preserve its integrity. Next, if indicated, the peroneal tendon sheath is incised longitu-dinally along the posterior fibula to allow exposure of the peroneal tendons (see **Fig. 7**B). In most cases, only a limited tenosynovectomy is required. After irrigation and closure of the peroneal tendon sheath with absorbable suture, the periosteal flap harvest is marked and lifted sharply off the lateral border of the fibula (see **Fig. 7**C–D). Next, the investigators release the capsuloligamentous complex from the lateral malleolus, identifying the ATFL remnant anteriorly (see **Fig. 7**E). Two small double-armed suture anchors (Arthrex, Naples, FL) are then placed in the distal fibula, approximately 1 to 2 cm proximal to the tip of the lateral malleolus. The suture anchors are placed in a parallel manner, at an angle 45° to the surface of the bone along the longitudinal axis of the fibula.

After placing the suture anchors, a 3-layered repair is performed. Using a small roll of surgical towels, the ankle is positioned in a neutral position, with the hindfoot in slight eversion. First, the capsuloligamentous complex is secured by passing the sutures through the leading edge of the tissue, advancing the complex retrograde over the lateral malleolus, and tying all 4 sutures from anterior to posterior (see **Fig. 7**F). We ensure that the ATFL remnant is captured in this first layer. We agree with previous investigators that it is not critical to incorporate the CFL in the repair.[17,21,35,71,83] Maintaining the same ankle-hindfoot position, the periosteal flap is advanced anterograde over the first layer of the repair and secured with the same sutures (see **Fig. 7**G). The IER is advanced to the repair site and secured by passing and securing all 4 sutures through its leading edge. The sutures are then cut, completing the repair (see **Fig. 7**H). The wound is irrigated and closed in a layered fashion. We routinely close the skin with interrupted mattress-type suture technique instead of metallic staples. Sterile dressings are applied, and a well-padded plaster splint is applied. The splint is applied with the ankle in neutral flexion and the hindfoot in subtle eversion to protect the ligamentous repair.

Concomitant Procedures

As discussed earlier, concomitant disease contributing to or resulting from chronic lateral ankle instability must be addressed at the time of any successful lateral liga-mentous reconstruction. Most commonly, these conditions include hindfoot malalign-ment, peroneal tendon diseases, and OCLTs.[18,19,51,52,88,89] Hindfoot varus or combined cavovarus deformities (see **Fig. 2**) are corrected with appropriate corrective osteotomies at the time of lateral ligament reconstruction. In addition, appropriate sur-gical procedures are performed to address peroneal tendinopathy(s) at the time of

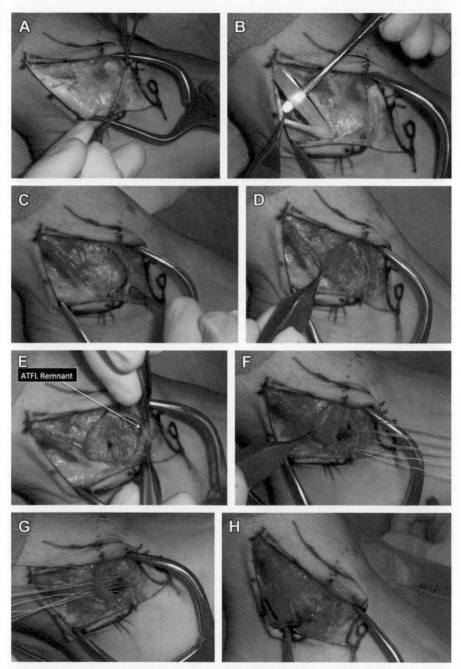

Fig. 7. (*A*) Intraoperative exposure and isolation of IER. (*B*) Exposure and exploration of normal-appearing peroneal tendons. (*C*) Marking of local distal fibular periosteal flap dissection for lateral ligamentous reconstruction augmentation. (*D*) Augmentative periosteal flap after subperiosteal dissection from lateral border of fibula. (*E*) Complete release of capsuloligamentous complex, exposing ATFL remnant. (*F*) Suture anchor repair of capsuloligamentous complex and ATFL remnant (layer 1). (*G*) Suture anchor repair of periosteal flap augmentation (layer 2). (*H*) Completed 3-layered lateral ligamentous reconstruction with periosteal flap augmentation.

lateral ligamentous reconstruction. If an OCLT is present (see **Fig. 1**), these are typically treated at the time of lateral ligamentous reconstruction with concomitant arthroscopic debridement and microfracture[18,19,88,89] or other indicated larger cartilage restorative procedures.

Postoperative Management

At our centers, all service members undergoing lateral ankle ligamentous reconstruction are evaluated preoperatively by physical therapists and are instructed to begin immediate postoperative hip and knee range of motion to minimize postoperative pain, swelling, thigh atrophy, and overall deconditioning. Service members then return to clinic at 2 weeks postoperatively for suture removal. The postoperative regimen is at the discretion of the individual surgeon and must be individually tailored to account for any other concomitant surgical procedures. In most cases, when only a standard primary lateral ligamentous repair with or without arthroscopy is performed, a weight-bearing short-leg fiberglass cast is placed at 2 weeks postoperatively. The patient is then allowed to begin weight bearing as tolerated. Generalized conditioning therapy continues, with the goal to prevent quadriceps atrophy and deconditioning. At 4 weeks postoperatively, the service member returns to clinic for removal of the cast and transition into a controlled ankle motion (CAM) boot for daily use. A structured postoperative functional rehabilitation program is initiated and tailored to the service member's individual needs, dependent on other concomitant procedures performed. During therapy sessions, the service member is allowed to remove the CAM boot and use a semirigid ankle brace (see **Fig. 6**). In addition, we allow service members to wear the brace at night during sleep.

In general, the rehabilitation course consists of 4 phases, incorporating a variety of lower extremity strengthening programs, seated and standing BAPS therapy to restore balance and proprioception, and focused peroneal tendon strengthening.[48,49,54,63,72,73] Between postoperative weeks 8 and 12, the CAM boot is discontinued and transition into a semirigid ankle brace is allowed at the therapist's discretion. A graduated walk to run program is generally initiated at the 12-week postoperative stage, and achievement of return to full sporting activities and military duties is expected by the 6-month postoperative stage. In military populations, we recommend using the semirigid ankle brace during running, sporting activities, and while on uneven surfaces until the 6-month postoperative stage. After 6 months, we allow service members to discontinue use of the brace altogether.

SUMMARY

Chronic lateral ankle instability is a condition frequently encountered by orthopedic surgeons treating highly active patient populations, particularly military service members. Providers treating military service members must have a high index of suspicion for this condition when signs and symptoms of functional or mechanical instability exist. Stress testing and ankle MRI, although not definitive in sensitivity for detecting instability or other concomitant injuries, should be considered during the treatment decision-making process. Appropriate nonoperative treatment should be attempted initially; however, when nonoperative treatment fails, surgical management is warranted to prevent untoward long-term sequelae. Proper surgical treatment and subsequent postoperative management are at the discretion of the individual surgeon but must account for the concomitant diseases frequently associated with chronic lateral ankle instability. Low recurrence of lateral instability can be achieved even in high-demand military patient populations with a focused treatment plan.

REFERENCES

1. Karlsson J, Sancone M. Management of acute ligament injuries of the ankle. Foot Ankle Clin 2006;11:521–30.
2. Kannus P, Renstrom P. Treatment for acute tears of the lateral ligaments of the ankle. Operation, cast, or early controlled mobilization. J Bone Joint Surg Am 1991;73:305–12.
3. Lynch SA, Renstrom PA. Treatment of acute lateral ankle ligament rupture in the athlete. Conservative versus surgical treatment. Sports Med 1999;27:61–71.
4. DiGiovanni CW, Brodsky A. Current concepts: lateral ankle instability. Foot Ankle Int 2006;27(10):854–66.
5. Colville M. Surgical treatment of the unstable ankle. J Am Acad Orthop Surg 1998;6:368–77.
6. DiGiovanni BF, Partal G, Baumhauer J. Acute ankle injury and chronic lateral instability in the athlete. Clin Sports Med 2004;23:1–19.
7. Barker HB, Beynnon BD, Renstrom PA. Ankle injury risk factors in sports. Sports Med 1997;23(2):69–74.
8. Garrick JG. The frequency of injury, mechanism of injury, and epidemiology of ankle sprains. Am J Sports Med 1977;5(6):241–2.
9. Gerber JP, Williams GN, Scoville CR, et al. Persistent disability with ankle sprains: a prospective examination of an athletic population. Foot Ankle Int 1998;19(10):653–60.
10. Malliaropoulos N, Ntessalen M, Papacostas E, et al. Reinjury after acute lateral ankle sprains in elite track and field athletes. Am J Sports Med 2009;37(9):1755–61.
11. Sitler MR, Ryan J, Wheeler B, et al. The efficacy of a semirigid ankle stabilizer to reduce acute ankle injuries in basketball: a randomized clinical study at West Point. Am J Sports Med 1994;22(4):454–61.
12. Kerkhoffs GM, Handoll HH, de Ble R, et al. Surgical versus conservative treatment for acute injuries of the lateral ligament complex of the ankle in adults. Cochrane Database Syst Rev 2002;(3):CD000380.
13. Pihlajamaki H, Hietaniemi K, Paavola M, et al. Surgical versus functional treatment for acute ruptures of the lateral ligament complex of the ankle in young men. J Bone Joint Surg Am 2010;92(14):2367–74.
14. Povacz P, Unger SF, Miller WK, et al. A randomized, prospective study of operative and non-operative treatment of injuries of the fibular collateral ligaments of the ankle. J Bone Joint Surg Am 1998;80:345–51.
15. Van Dijk CN. Management of the sprained ankle. Br J Sports Med 2002;36:83–4.
16. Berlet G, Anderson RB, Davis W. Chronic lateral ankle instability. Foot Ankle Clin 1999;4:713–28.
17. Li X, Killie H, Guerrero P, et al. Anatomical reconstruction for chronic lateral ankle instability in the high-demand athlete. Am J Sports Med 2009;37(3):487–94.
18. Sugimoto K, Takakura Y, Okahashi K, et al. Chondral injuries of the ankle with recurrent lateral instability: an arthroscopic study. J Bone Joint Surg Am 2009; 91:99–106.
19. Ferkel RD, Chams RN. Chronic lateral instability: arthroscopic findings and long-term results. Foot Ankle Int 2007;28(1):24–31.
20. Heckman DS, Reddy S, Pedowitz D, et al. Operative treatment for peroneal tendon disorders. J Bone Joint Surg Am 2008;90(2):404–18.
21. Maffulli N, Del Buono A, Maffulli GD, et al. Isolated anterior talofibular ligament Broström repair for chronic lateral ankle instability. 9-year follow-up. Am J Sports Med 2013;41(4):858–64.

22. Maffulli N, Ferran NA. Management of acute and chronic ankle instability. J Am Acad Orthop Surg 2008;16(10):608–15.
23. Kennedy JG, Brunner JB, Bohne WH, et al. Clinical importance of the lateral branch of the deep peroneal nerve. Clin Orthop Relat Res 2007;459:222–8.
24. Orr JD, Dawson LK, Garcia EJ, et al. Incidence of osteochondral lesions of the talus in the United States military. Foot Ankle Int 2011;32(10):948–54.
25. Waterman BR, Belmont PJ Jr, Cameron KL, et al. Epidemiology of ankle sprain at the United States Military Academy. Am J Sports Med 2010;38(4):797–803.
26. Burks RT, Morgan J. Anatomy of the lateral ankle ligaments. Am J Sports Med 1994;22:72–7.
27. Ferran NA, Maffulli N. Epidemiology of sprains of the lateral ankle ligament complex. Foot Ankle Clin 2006;11:659–62.
28. Lofvenberg R, Karrholm J, Ahlgren O, et al. Prolonged reaction time in patients with chronic lateral instability of the ankle. Am J Sports Med 1995;23:414–7.
29. O'Loughlin PF, Hodgkins CW, Kennedy JG. Ankle sprains and instability in dancers. Clin Sports Med 2008;27:247–62.
30. Attarian DE, Meerackin HJ, Devito DP, et al. Biomechanical characteristics of human ankle ligaments. Foot Ankle 1985;6:54–7.
31. Stephens MM, Sammarco GJ. The stabilizing role of the lateral complex around the ankle and subtalar joints. Foot Ankle 1992;13:130–6.
32. Bulucu C, Thomas KA, Halvorson TL, et al. Biomechanical evaluation of the anterior drawer test: the contribution of the lateral ankle ligaments. Foot Ankle Int 1991;11:389–93.
33. Hintermann B. Biomechanics of the unstable ankle joint and clinical applications. Med Sci Sports Exerc 1999;31(7 Suppl):S459–69.
34. Broström L. Sprained ankles. I. Anatomic lesions in recent sprains. Acta Chir Scand 1964;128:483–95.
35. Broström L. Sprained ankles. VI. Surgical treatment of "chronic" ligament ruptures. Acta Chir Scand 1966;132:551–65.
36. Hirose K, Murakami G, Minowa T, et al. Lateral ligament injury of the ankle and associated articular cartilage degeneration in the talocrural joint: anatomic study using elderly cadavers. J Orthop Sci 2004;9:37–43.
37. Renstrom P, Wertz M, Incavo S, et al. Strain in the lateral ligaments of the ankle. Foot Ankle 1988;9:59–63.
38. Hertel J. Functional anatomy, pathomechanics, and pathophysiology of lateral ankle instability. J Athl Train 2002;37:364–75.
39. Waterman BR, Langston JR, Cameron KL, et al. Sprain in the forecast. Epidemiology and risk factors for ankle sprain. Lower Extremity Review. 2011. Available at: http://lowerextremityreview.com/cover_story/sprain-in-the-forecast-epidemiology-and-risk-factors-for-ankle-sprain. Accessed January 9, 2014.
40. Waterman BR, Owens BD, Davey S, et al. The epidemiology of ankle sprain in the United States. J Bone Joint Surg Am 2010;92(13):2279–84.
41. Frey C, Feder KS, Sleight J. Prophylactic ankle brace use in high school volleyball players. A prospective study. Foot Ankle Int 2010;31(4):296–300.
42. Heitz NA, Eisenman PA, Beck CL, et al. Hormonal changes throughout the menstrual cycle and increased anterior cruciate ligament laxity in females. J Athl Train 1999;34(2):144–9.
43. Huston LJ, Greenfield ML, Wojtys EM. Anterior cruciate ligament injuries in the female athlete: potential risk factors. Clin Orthop Relat Res 2000;(372):50–63.
44. Department of the Army. Women in the US Army. Available at: http://www.army.mil/women/today.html. Accessed January 10, 2014.

45. Cameron KL. Time for a paradigm shift in conceptualizing risk factors in sports injury research. J Athl Train 2010;45(1):58–60.
46. Tyler TF, McHugh MP, Mirabella MR, et al. Risk factors for noncontact ankle sprains in high school football players: the role of previous ankle sprains and body mass index. Am J Sports Med 2006;34(3):471–5.
47. Holmer P, Sondergaard L, Konradsen L, et al. Epidemiology of sprains in the lateral ankle and foot. Foot Ankle Int 1994;15:72–4.
48. Rosenbaum D, Eils E. A multistation proprioceptive exercise program in patients with ankle instability. Med Sci Sports Exerc 2001;33:1991–8.
49. Frank C, Amiel D, Woo SL, et al. Normal ligament properties and ligament healing. Clin Orthop Relat Res 1985;(196):15–25.
50. McGuine TA, Greene JJ, Best T, et al. Balance as a predictor of ankle injuries in high school basketball players. Clin Sports Med 2000;10(4):239–44.
51. Fortin PT, Guettler J, Manoli A II. Idiopathic cavovarus and lateral ankle instability: recognition and treatment implications relating to ankle arthritis. Foot Ankle Int 2002;23(11):1031–7.
52. Larsen E, Angermann P. Association of ankle instability and foot deformity. Acta Orthop Scand 1990;61(2):136–9.
53. Freeman MA, Dean MR, Hanham IW. The etiology and prevention of functional instability of the foot. J Bone Joint Surg Br 1965;47(4):678–85.
54. Leanderson J, Eriksson E, Nilsson C, et al. Proprioception in classical ballet dancers. A prospective study of the influence of an ankle sprain on proprioception in the ankle joint. Am J Sports Med 1996;24(3):370–4.
55. Leanderson J, Wykman A, Eriksson E. Ankle sprain and postural sway in basketball players. Knee Surg Sports Traumatol Arthrosc 1993;1(3-4):203–5.
56. Perrin PP, Bene MC, Perrin CA, et al. Ankle trauma significantly impairs posture control. A study in basketball players and controls. Int J Sports Med 1997;18(5):387–92.
57. Trojian TH, McKeag DB. Single leg balance test to identify risk of ankle sprains. Br J Sports Med 2006;40(7):610–3.
58. Grahame R, Bird HA, Child A. The revised (Brighton 1998) criteria for the diagnosis of BJHS. J Rheumatol 2000;27:1777–9.
59. Cerrato RA, Myerson MS. Peroneal tendon tears, surgical management and its complications. Foot Ankle Clin 2009;14(2):299–312.
60. Maffulli N. Recurrent subluxation of the peroneal tendons. Am J Sports Med 2006;34(6):986–92.
61. Laurin CA, Ouellet R, St-Jacques R. Talar and subtalar tilt: an experimental investigation. Can J Surg 1968;11:270–9.
62. Fugii T, Luo ZP, Kitaoka HB, et al. The manual stress test may not be sufficient to differentiate ankle ligament injuries. J Biomech 2000;15:619–23.
63. Matsuaka N, Yokoyama S, Tsursaki T, et al. Effect of ankle disk training combined with tactile stimulation to the leg and foot on functional instability of the ankle. Am J Sports Med 2001;29:25–30.
64. Boyle J, Negus V. Joint position sense in the recurrently sprained ankle. Aust J Physiother 1998;44:159–63.
65. Tropp H, Odernick P, Gilguist J. Stabilometry recordings in functional and mechanical instability of the ankle joint. Int J Sports Med 1985;6:180–2.
66. Larsen E. Static or dynamic repair of chronic lateral ankle instability. A prospective randomized study. Clin Orthop Relat Res 1990;(257):184–92.
67. Rosenbaum D, Engelhardt M, Becker HP, et al. Clinical and functional outcome after anatomic and nonanatomic ankle ligament reconstruction: Evans tenodesis versus periosteal flap. Foot Ankle Int 1999;20:636–9.

68. O'Neill PJ, Van Aman SE, Guyton GP. Is MRI adequate to detect lesions in patients with ankle instability? Clin Orthop Relat Res 2010;468(4):1115–9.
69. DiGiovanni BF, Fraga CJ, Cohen BE, et al. Associated injuries found in chronic lateral ankle instability. Foot Ankle Int 2000;21:809–15.
70. Frey C. Ankle sprains. Instr Course Lect 2001;50:515–20.
71. Ng ZD, De SD. Modified Broström-Evans-Gould technique for recurrent ankle lateral ligament instability. J Orthop Surg 2007;15(3):306–10.
72. Hoffman M, Payne VG. The effects of proprioceptive ankle disk training on healthy subjects. J Orthop Sports Phys Ther 1995;21(2):90–3.
73. Tropp H, Askling C, Gillquist J. Prevention of ankle sprains. Am J Sports Med 1985;13:259–62.
74. Ajis A, Maffulli N. Conservative management of chronic ankle instability. Foot Ankle Clin 2006;11:531–7.
75. Rovere GD, Clarke TJ, Yates CS, et al. Retrospective comparison of taping and ankle stabilizers in preventing ankle injuries. Am J Sports Med 1988;16:228–33.
76. Karlsson J, Bergsten T, Lansinger O, et al. Surgical treatment of chronic lateral instability of the ankle joint. A new procedure. Am J Sports Med 1989;17:268–73.
77. Karlsson J, Ericksson B, Bergsten T, et al. Comparison of two anatomic reconstructions for chronic lateral instability of the ankle. Am J Sports Med 1997;25:48–53.
78. Ayogdan U, Glisson RR, Nunley JA. Extensor retinaculum augmentation reinforces anterior talofibular ligament repair. Clin Orthop Relat Res 2006;442:210–5.
79. Waldrop NE, Wijdicks CA, Jansson KS, et al. Anatomic suture anchor versus the Broström technique for anterior talofibular ligament repair. Am J Sports Med 2012;40(11):2590–6.
80. Messer TM, Cummins CA, Ahn J, et al. Outcome of the modified Broström procedure for chronic lateral ankle instability using suture anchors. Foot Ankle Int 2000;21:996–1003.
81. Okazaki K, Miyagi S, Tokunaga J. Anatomic reconstruction of the lateral ligament of the ankle using a periosteal flap from the fibula. Tech Foot Ankle Surg 2005;4:98–103.
82. Kirk KL, Schon LC. Technique tip: periosteal flap augmentation of the Broström lateral ankle reconstruction. Foot Ankle Int 2008;29(2):254–5.
83. Bell SJ, Mologne TS, Sitler DF, et al. Twenty-six year results after Broström procedure for chronic lateral ankle instability. Am J Sports Med 2006;34:975–8.
84. Korkala O, Sorvali T. Twenty year results of the Evans operation for lateral instability of the ankle. Clin Orthop Relat Res 2002;(405):195–8.
85. Rosenbaum D, Becker H, Sterk J, et al. Functional evaluation of 10-year outcome after modified Evans repair for chronic ankle instability. Foot Ankle Int 1997;18:765–71.
86. Colville M, Grondel RJ. Anatomic reconstruction of the lateral ankle ligaments using a split peroneus brevis tendon graft. Am J Sports Med 1995;23:210–3.
87. Solakoglu C, Kiral AL, Pehlivan O. Late-term reconstruction of the lateral ankle ligaments using a split peroneus brevis graft (Colville technique) in patients with chronic lateral instability of the ankle. Int Orthop 2003;27:223–7.
88. Komenda GA, Ferkel RD. Arthroscopic findings associated with the unstable ankle. Foot Ankle Int 1999;20:708–13.
89. Van Dijk CN, Bossuyt PM, Marti RK. Medial ankle pain after lateral ligament rupture. J Bone Joint Surg Br 1996;78:562–7.
90. Glas E, Paar O, Samsal B, et al. Periosteal flap reconstruction of the external ankle ligaments: results of a follow-up study. Unfallchirurg 1985;88:219–22.

Chronic Exertional Compartment Syndrome of the Leg in the Military

John C. Dunn, MD[a], Brian R. Waterman, MD[a,b,c],*

KEYWORDS

- Chronic exertional compartment syndrome • Intracompartmental pressure
- Paresthesia

KEY POINTS

- Chronic exertional compartment syndrome affects young athletic individuals, especially those in active duty military service.
- Nonoperative treatment may benefit low-demand patients; however, in an athletic cohort surgical decompression must be considered in a patient that fails conservative management.
- Although good surgical outcomes have been reported by tertiary referral centers, return to duty rates in the military are poor, with only 55% of patients experiencing complete resolution of symptoms.
- Patient education, activity modification, and gait retraining may be beneficial to optimize symptomatic relief.

INTRODUCTION

Activity-related lower extremity pain is common among athletes and other active patient populations. Along with other overuse conditions, chronic exertional compartment syndrome (CECS) may contribute significantly to the development of effort-dependent leg symptoms. One of the earliest descriptions of CECS occurred during the British expedition to the South Pole in 1912, in which Edward Wilson described anterior leg swelling and pain during long treks in the Arctic.[1] Subsequent historical records have also emphasized the prevalence of CECS in military cohorts,[2,3] earning the appellation "march gangrene."[4]

Conflict of Interest: None.
The opinions or assertions contained herein are the private views of the authors and are not to be construed as official or reflecting the views of the Department of Defense or the US government. The authors are employees of the US government.
[a] Department of Orthopaedic Surgery and Rehabilitation, William Beaumont Army Medical Center, 5005 North Piedras Street, El Paso, TX 79920-5001, USA; [b] Department of Orthopaedic Surgery, Texas Tech University Health Sciences Center, El Paso, Texas; [c] Uniformed Services University of Health Sciences, Bethesda, Maryland
* Corresponding author.
E-mail address: brian.r.waterman@gmail.com

Clin Sports Med 33 (2014) 693–705
http://dx.doi.org/10.1016/j.csm.2014.06.010
0278-5919/14/$ – see front matter Published by Elsevier Inc.
sportsmed.theclinics.com

Acute compartment syndrome typically develops after trauma, and secondary tissue ischemia and muscle breakdown warrant emergent fasciotomy to preserve limb viability. By contrast, CECS, otherwise known as exercise-induced compartment syndrome, develops after prolonged exertion in the absence of injury and it is often evaluated in the ambulatory setting. During intensive exercise, intramuscular volume can expand by up to 20% in response to increased metabolic demands, tissue perfusion, and muscle fiber hypertrophy.[5–7] When sustained, compartment syndrome may develop as the interstitial pressure becomes critically elevated above the diastolic pressure of a closed fascial compartment. Consequently, compromised vascular perfusion leads to tissue ischemia, metabolite accumulation, and extremity pain. Alternatively, other investigators have proposed that fluid extravasation and increased intracompartmental pressures (ICPs) contribute to neural compression and potentially irreversible damage with chronic untreated compartment syndrome. Other investigators have also implicated decreased capillary density or hindered venous outflow in the development of CECS.[8,9]

Although the pathophysiology is not fully understood, CECS remains a frequent source of lower extremity disability in contemporary military service members. With heightened occupational demands, daily exercise, and mandated physical fitness performance standards, the military represents a unique, high-demand population at elevated risk for the development of CECS. This article explores the epidemiology, risk factors, diagnosis, and management of CECS within this cohort.

EPIDEMIOLOGY AND RISK FACTORS

The exact prevalence of CECS is currently unclear because of the frequency of self-directed treatment or activity modification, errors in clinical diagnosis, and/or failure to seek medical attention. According to smaller series, CECS may account for 14% to 34% of activity-related leg pain referred for orthopedic treatment.[10–12] Further estimates have indicated that approximately one in every 2000 US military service members is diagnosed with CECS each year,[13] with 4100 individuals identified over a 6-year period.

CECS is most commonly described in the leg, accounting for more than 95% of all cases.[14] However, other investigators have variably reported involvement of the hand,[15,16] forearm,[17–19] thigh,[20,21] and foot[22] in narrow high-risk cohorts. When evaluating the distribution of CECS in the compartments of the leg, the anterior compartment is most frequently affected (42%–60%) followed by the lateral (35%–36%), deep posterior (19%–32%), and the superficial posterior (3%–21%).[10,23] Davis and colleagues[23] found that single compartment involvement was less common (37%). In their series, 40% of cases were symptomatic in two compartments, 18% involved three compartments, and only 5% affected all four compartments. Similarly, bilateral involvement is more common, accounting for up to 95%[23,24] and no differences by laterality have previously been identified.[25]

This condition has usually been described among younger, athletic populations. Patients typically present in the second and early fourth decade of life, often with a long duration of preexisting symptoms.[23,26,27] Earlier studies have described a greater preponderance of affected men,[8,12,28] whereas other investigations have suggested the potential for increased incidence among women.[9,13,23] Meanwhile, selected investigations from the civilian literature have reported that the incidence of CECS between men and women is roughly equal.[10,11,26]

More than 90% of patients presenting with CECS are involved in athletics[23] and there is no reported difference between those involved in elite and recreational levels of competition.[5] Although many forms of athletics have been linked with the development of CECS of the leg, including lacrosse, soccer, basketball, skiing, and field hockey,[23] it is most characteristically described in endurance runners,[5,12,23] which accounts for up to 68% of cases.[26] However, CECS may also present in less-active, atypical patient populations. Edmundsson and colleagues[9] reported on a series of 36 nonathletic, more sedentary subjects with CECS. In this cohort, nearly two-thirds of subjects developed pain after routine walking and low-demand activity.

Excessive exercise, especially running, has been linked to increased incidence of CECS.[23] Significant physical activity precipitates physiologic and metabolic changes that affect muscle volume and compartment pressures.[5-7] Eccentric muscle strengthening in adults has been implicated as a cause for decreased fascial compliance and the development of CECS.[29] Similarly, patients with CECS have been found to have a thickened fascia[30] and may have a higher prevalence of fascial defects compared with asymptomatic patients.[31] These factors can also be exacerbated by dietary supplements. The use of muscle enhancing supplements, such as creatine and androgenic steroids, may potentiate abnormal elevations in ICPs, and these have been offered as possible risk factors for CECS.[5]

As with other active cohorts, CECS is commonly reported among military populations[1-4,13,25,32] and should be separately considered due to its unique occupational demands. Recently published, large-scale reviews of this military subset have underscored the burden of lower extremity CECS among this high-risk cohort.[13,25] In this study, although greater than 90% of subjects with CECS were men, women had a slightly higher incidence rate while controlling for other variables. Similarly, junior enlisted military rank and Army service carried the highest incidence rate of developing CECS, which is likely attributable to the increased physical rigors of ground forces in the current military conflicts. Interestingly, increasing age category corresponded with increasing incidence rates of CECS in the military. This may reflect a previously undetected association between age and the development of CECS and certainly merits further investigation.

CLINICAL PRESENTATION AND DIAGNOSIS

In terms of frequency, CECS is the second-leading cause of exertional leg pain after medial tibial stress syndrome (MTSS), with a prevalence of up to one-third of athletes.[10] The differential diagnosis should also include evaluations for nerve entrapment, stress fracture, deep vein thrombosis, and other clinical entities (**Table 1**). The natural history of CECS is mostly atraumatic, although a remote history of low-energy injury may be disclosed in certain individuals.[33] Patients often complain of tightness, pain, or aching in the anterior and lateral portion of the leg after periods of prolonged exercise, and these symptoms often resolve with rest or diminished activity. As previously mentioned, symptoms are bilateral in up to 95% of patients.[24] In addition to neuritic symptoms overlying the superficial peroneal nerve distribution, affected patients may also show decreased vibratory sensation and altered motor amplitude that contribute to poor foot and ankle control.[34]

History and physical examination are the cornerstones for a diagnosis of CECS. It is important to document the frequency, duration, and intensity of training sessions, as well as corresponding trends in onset and resolution of patient-reported symptoms. At rest, the patient may not have any symptoms; however, on exertion the patient may develop significant activity-limiting symptoms. Patients with CECS typically complain of five cardinal symptoms: pain, tightness, cramps, weakness, and diminished sensibility in the dorsum of the foot.[35] On physical examination, pain on passive stretch of a

Table 1
Sources of leg pain in physically-active patients

Category	Condition	Diagnosis
Vascular	Popliteal artery entrapment syndrome	Ankle or brachial index, Doppler
	Popliteal artery aneurysm	Angiogram
	Deep vein thrombosis	Doppler
Bone	Tibial stress fracture	MRI
	Medial tibial stress syndrome	Bone scintigraphy
	Periostalgia	Infection work-up
Soft Tissue	Muscle strain	Physical examination
	Tendinopathy	—
	Tenosynovitis	—
	CECS	ICP, MRI, near-infrared spectroscopy
Neurologic	Peripheral nerve entrapment (superficial peroneal nerve, tibial nerve)	Electromyogram, nerve conduction studies
	Neurogenic claudication	—
Miscellaneous	Metabolic bone disease	Dual energy x-ray absorptiometry
	Muscle or bone neoplasm	MRI
	Bone or soft tissue infection	—

compartment may be present if the patient has recently exercised, although this would be rare at rest. Fascial defects may also be detected on palpation and are present in 39% to 46% of affected patients.[6–10]

Although currently debated, the historical standard for diagnosis of CECS has been ICP measurement.[36] ICP monitoring may be completed with many commercial devices.[36] At the authors' institution, the Stryker Intra-Compartmental Monitor (Stryker Corporation, Kalamazoo, MI, USA) is commonly used as a component of the standard preoperative evaluation, with comparison of affected and unaffected compartments in bilateral lower extremities (**Fig. 1**). On presentation, patients complete an exercise stress test. A series of manometry measurements are taken both before and after exercise to analyze ICP trends of symptomatic compartments. Typical resting ICPs of the leg measures less than 10 mm Hg, although measurements are operator-dependent and may vary considerably between patients.[36]

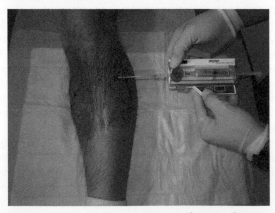

Fig. 1. ICPs measurements of the leg for evaluation of CECS after exercise stress testing. (*Courtesy of* Justin Orr, MD, El Paso, TX.)

Davis and colleagues[23] carefully monitored a cohort of CECS subjects during exercise stress testing. In this analysis, subjects reported having leg pain after an average of 11 minutes of exertion. The exertional leg pain was rated as an eight out of ten on the visual analog scale, and symptoms subsided after an average of 45 minutes of rest. In this study, 36% of the subjects developed numbness or tingling in addition to pain after exertion. CECS was also objectively quantified after exercise testing. The anterior compartment increased from a preexercise average of 25.3 mm Hg to an average of 48 mm Hg after exercise stress testing, with similarly increased readings in the lateral (baseline 21.5 to 51.5 mm Hg postexercise), deep posterior (22.1 to 47.1 mm Hg), and superficial posterior compartments (24.9 to 34.3 mm Hg).

As an adjunct to clinical examination, Pedowitz and colleagues[10] established several diagnostic criteria to confirm the presence of CECS. If one of these three criteria is met, a diagnosis of CECS may be made: (1) a preexercise pressure of greater than 15 mm Hg, (2) a 1-minute postexercise pressure of greater than 30 mm Hg, or (3) a 5-minute post-exercise pressure of greater than 20 mm Hg. Although these thresholds are the most widely used in current clinical practice, pressure measurements are not always reliable and may be confounded by poor patient tolerance, inconsistent operator technique, and/or the use of different measurement devices. To this end, Aweid and colleagues[36] reviewed 32 studies that evaluated the usefulness of ICP measurements in the diagnosis of CECS. Reported preexercise ICPs ranged from 7.4 to 50.8 mm Hg in CECS subjects and 5.7 to 12 mm Hg in controls, whereas postexercise measurements ranged from 42 to 150 mm Hg and 28 to 141 mm Hg, respectively. At 1-minute postexercise, there was less overlap between subjects with CECS and controls (CECS, 34–55.4 mm Hg; controls, 9–19 mm Hg). The investigators concluded that there is limited evidence to validate four commonly used criteria using ICPs for the evaluation of patients with lower extremity pain. Furthermore, they suggested that a diagnosis of CECS should rely more heavily on classic clinical presentation.

In addition to ICP monitoring, other modalities may hold promise for diagnosis of CECS. Although not commonly used in current practice, the use of MRI has been reported and may useful in excluding other disease, such as MTSS.[37] Postexercise MRI has demonstrated increased diffuse intracompartmental signal on T2 sequences when compared with baseline and this may be pronounced in symptomatic patients.[37,38] Although these studies examined the increase in intracompartmental edema, MRI can also be scrutinized for fascial defects or other structural lesions. With that said, the use of MRI is not well studied in the setting of CECS and would likely prove logistically difficult after exercise stress testing. The use of near-infrared spectroscopy (NIRS) has recently been studied in Europe as a measure of oxygen saturation of hemoglobin in deep tissues. Although less well studied than direct intracompartmental measurement, NIRS offers a noninvasive technique with improved patient tolerance. van den Brand and colleagues[39] evaluated subjects after an exercise test with NIRS and demonstrated a significant decrease in oxygen saturation in patients with CECS compared with controls. When compared with other diagnostic modalities,[40] NIRS was at least as efficacious as MRI or ICP monitoring for patients with known CECS. The sensitivity of ICP monitoring was 77%, 85% for NIRS, and 86% for MRI. Although MRI and NIRS have potential as noninvasive tools in the diagnosis of CECS, ICP monitoring remains the most prevalent.

NONSURGICAL TREATMENT

The reported results of nonoperative management are modest and conservative interventions have generally been unsuccessful in restoring active patients to pain-free physical activity. In a retrospective cohort study comparing nonoperative and surgical management of CECS, Packer and colleagues[41] reported that only 41% of subjects experienced significant symptomatic relief with activity modification, ice, medication, and/or physical therapy. These and other specific modalities to alleviate symptoms, including massage, orthotics, and stretching, have been associated inconsistent outcomes and incomplete relief.[29,42] Blackman and colleagues[42] demonstrated significant delays in the onset of pain during athletic activity after a 5-week stretching and massage regimen. However, ICP measurements remained unchanged, and most subjects had persisting complaints of exertional leg pain. Activity limitation remains the single most effective measure to reduce symptomatic episodes.[32] Running may be substituted with cycling or other forms of aerobic exercises to maintain cardiorespiratory fitness because these alternatives have been associated with a lower risk of CECS.[43] However, complete avoidance of exercise is not an option for many patients involved in competitive athletics or endurance running. Similarly, although daily physical fitness routines can be customized to mitigate symptoms, certain at-risk activities (eg, ruck marching, training exercises) associated with military service cannot be curtailed.

Recent research has suggested that alterations in running biomechanics and tailored physical therapy protocols may be beneficial in selected individuals with CECS. In a cadet cohort at the US Military Academy, a forefoot running program was initiated for 10 symptomatic subjects with a hindfoot strike gait pattern and indications for surgical intervention (**Fig. 2**).[44] The underlying premise is that a forefoot running technique diminishes the increased ICP and eccentric activity of the anterior compartment while reducing ground-reaction forces. After intervention, all subjects demonstrated significant improvements in running performance and exercise-induced pain, with sustained benefits indicated on subject-reported outcome measures at up to 1 year. More importantly, the average postexercise ICP decreased from 78 mm Hg to 32 mm Hg after 6 weeks of forefoot running training and all patients avoided surgical treatment. A large-scale, prospective, randomized trial is warranted to determine the comparative efficacy of gait retraining vis-à-vis elective surgical intervention.

SURGICAL TREATMENT

When nonsurgical measures are ineffective or patients are unwilling to accept permanent activity or duty restrictions, operative management may be considered, with decompression of all symptomatic compartments. Although, historically, most investigators have described fasciotomy for elective treatment of CECS, selective use of partial fasciectomy for primary[45] or revision cases[46] may also be considered.

For isolated anterior, lateral, or combined anterolateral involvement, a single lateral incision may be used. The single incision technique involves a longitudinal incision from just anterior and proximal to the lateral malleolus and extends to the fibular neck. The lateral and anterior compartments are identified in relation to the intermuscular septum. These are then released by making an "H" in the fascia with Metzenbaum scissors. After identifying the superficial peroneal nerve, the fascial release is taken distally and proximally in each anterior and lateral compartment. Owing to the presence of anomalous neural anatomy and the risk of iatrogenic neural injury during fasciotomy, the authors prefer a more limited, distally-based incision overlying the exit of the superficial peroneal nerve at the intermuscular fascia (**Fig. 3**). When neuritic symptoms predominate, we also recommend careful neurolysis of the superficial peroneal nerve and scrutiny for any potential sites for scar tissue entrapment.

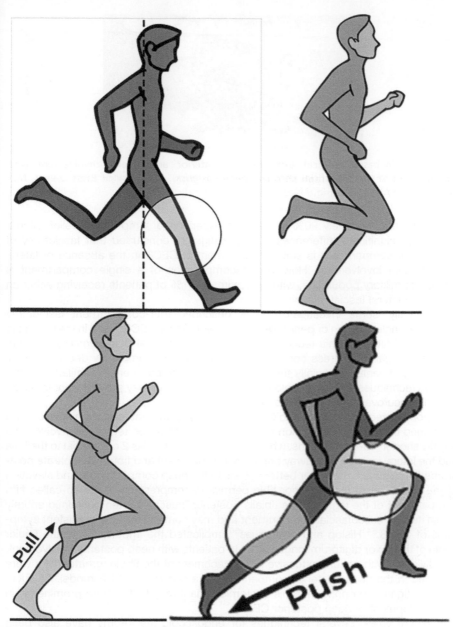

Fig. 2. Physical therapy and gait retraining emphasizing a transition from a hindfoot to a forefoot strike method for the treatment of anterior CECS. (*Courtesy of* Pose Tech, Inc, Miami, FL; with permission.)

Decompression of a single anterior compartment without adjacent lateral compartment release has previously been a topic of debate. In a prospective comparative investigation, Schepsis and colleagues[47] performed fasciotomies on subjects with bilateral leg CECS in which one leg received anterior and lateral compartment decompression and the contralateral leg underwent isolated anterior release. Regardless of

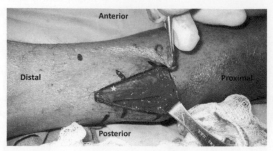

Fig. 3. Distally-based surgical exposure for anterior and lateral involvement with identification of the superficial peroneal nerve (*asterisk*). (*Courtesy of* Brett Owens, MD, West Point, NY.)

technique, approximately 90% of subjects experienced symptomatic relief without statistically significant differences. The investigators concluded that fasciotomy of the anterior compartment is sufficient treatment of CECS in the absence of lateral compartment involvement. However, decompression of a single compartment is rare in the military population, with approximately 1% of patients receiving either an anterior or lateral fascial release.

Historically, some investigators have described four-compartment fasciotomy through a single-incision or perifibular technique, both for CECS[31] and in the traumatic setting.[48–50] Although this technique obviates an additional posteromedial incision, some investigators express concern about the ability to completely decompress all four compartments, especially the deep posterior compartment.[51] Similarly, single-incision techniques also may prolong operative times and may provide poorer visualization of neurovascular structures at risk.

As popularized by Mubarak and Owen,[52] four-compartment fasciotomy can also be performed through a dual-incision technique.[53] This preferred technique involves two slightly shorter, 10-cm incisions, where the medial incision lies 2 cm medial to the tibia and the lateral incision is midway between the tibial crest and fibula. A separate posteromedial approach may offer better access to the deep compartments and elevation of the soleus off of the posterior tibia permits decompression of the so-called fifth compartment of the leg.[54,55] The tibialis posterior muscle is often contained entirely within its own osseofascial compartment and may contribute to the persistent symptoms of CECS.[54] Hislop and colleagues[56] implicated the importance of the fibular origin of the flexor digitorum longus (FDL) in patients with deep posterior involvement. In individuals with a more extensive FDL attachment at the fibula, greater ICPs were detected in the deep posterior compartment in a cadaveric CECS model. As such, the investigators propose that this anatomic variant may factor more prominently in the development of deep posterior CECS.

In recent years, several techniques for endoscopic fasciotomy have also been described, with encouraging results in multiple, small case series.[57–61] This offers a minimally-invasive approach with improved cosmesis and the potential for less postoperative scar formation. Advocates have also noted excellent visualization of the intermuscular septum, superficial peroneal nerve, and perforating vessels without use of a traditional incision. However, these investigations are of limited enrollment and are best suited for isolated anterolateral involvement.

After meticulous hemostasis and wound closure with a two-compartment or four-compartment fasciotomy, a standardized physical therapy protocol is undertaken. At our military institution, knee and ankle range of motion exercises and gentle scar mobilization are initiated early to prevent fascial adhesions. Staged fasciotomy (greater than 6 weeks) for patients with bilateral involvement is recommended, although concurrent intervention may be considered for selected, motivated patients. Patients are instructed for touch-down weight-bearing with crutches for 4 weeks, with progression to full weight-bearing as tolerated by week six. Thereafter, patients begin a progressive strengthening program and may begin walking on a treadmill. By the twelfth week, patients may begin a transition to running program. At 4-months post-operatively, the goal is to pass the Army Physical Fitness Test. This protocol has been successfully used in war zones[62] and is also similar to that described for the civilian populations.[63]

In reported civilian cohorts, the results of surgical treatment of CECS are generally encouraging, with up to 90% to 96% of patients reporting good to excellent outcomes.[12,26,64] However, the treatment of patients with posterior involvement is much less reliable than that for isolated anterior CECS. In one study, release of the anterior compartments resulted in 96% excellent results, whereas the release of the posterior compartments yielded only 25% excellent results.[64] Other published data have reported an 80% success rate for anterior and lateral releases, whereas only 50% of subjects with fasciotomy of the posterior compartments experience significant relief.[27] The cause of this is not well elucidated, although thickened posterior fascia and scar formation have been proposed.[26] Additionally, inadequate decompression of all deep posterior compartments may also compromise surgical outcomes, particularly with limited release of the soleus and deep posterior compartments. To this end, Rorabeck and colleagues[53] have suggested that formally releasing the tibialis posterior may improve outcomes of the posterior fasciotomy. More aggressive decompression using partial fasciectomy has not demonstrated any increased usefulness versus traditional fasciotomy in index procedures for CECS, with only 60% successful outcomes after release.[45]

Although the civilian literature has reported beneficial results, the clinical outcomes after surgical release in the military population have been less optimal for CECS of the leg. In a review of 611 US military service members with 754 surgical releases, 78% of patients were free from medical discharge or revision after index surgery at short-term to mid-term follow-up.[25] These results parallel the 73% success rate reported by Almdahl and Samdal[65] in the Norwegian military. However, 28% of service members were unable to return to full duty in the US military cohort and 45% experienced incomplete relief of symptoms.[25] In similar study of UK military personnel with CECS, only 47% of subjects' symptoms improved after surgery.[66] Presumably, these poor outcomes are partially attributable to the rigorous daily physical fitness demands common to the military.

PERIOPERATIVE COMPLICATIONS AND REVISION SURGERY

Perioperative complications often manifest early after surgical intervention, most commonly with local surgical site infections, wound healing difficulties, hematoma or seroma development, and/or iatrogenic neurovascular injury. By contrast, recurrences typically occur after an initial symptom-free interval, and may result from inadequate release, failure to decompress a symptomatic compartment, postsurgical fibrosis, or nerve compression. Entrapment of the superficial peroneal nerve has been found in 44% of subjects presenting with recurrent CECS after initial surgical treatment and remains an important consideration during primary and revision procedures.[46] In subjects with localized neuritic symptoms, Schepsis and colleagues[46] demonstrated 100% satisfactory outcomes with partial fasciectomy, decompression of the superficial peroneal nerve, and excision of all fibrotic tissue during revision surgery. Conversely, all subjects without nerve entrapment had a 50% success rate after revision surgery.

Whereas prior civilian series have documented complications in up to 11%[26] and recurrence in 2% to 17%,[12,27,53,64] military cohorts have demonstrated a higher risk of adverse surgical outcomes.[25,66] In a Norwegian military cohort with 10-year follow-up on 56 fascial releases for anterior compartment CECS, 2% of subjects required repeat fasciotomy.[65] Another contemporary analysis involving the US military revealed a complication rate of 15.7% after elective fasciotomies for CECS.[25] In this case series, nearly three-quarter of these were identified as infections or other wound-healing problems, whereas approximately 25% were related to neurologic injury. Furthermore, the rate of surgical revision was 5.9%, with 14% of service members experiencing complete resolution of symptoms and 67% returning to full activity. Finally, an evaluation of the UK military population revealed that infection was also the most common complication (9%), followed by seroma and hematoma formation.[66]

SUMMARY

CECS is a common source of lower extremity disability among young athletic cohorts and military personnel. The five cardinal symptoms are pain, tightness, cramps, weakness, and diminished sensation. History and clinical examination remain the hallmarks for identifying CECS, although ICP measurements during exercise stress testing may be used to confirm diagnosis. Nonsurgical management is generally unsuccessful, although gait retraining may have benefits in selected individuals. When conservative measures have failed, operative management may be considered with fascial release of all affected compartments. Although clinical success has been documented in civilian cohorts, the results of surgical treatment in military service members have been far less reliable. Only approximately half of the military service members experience complete resolution of symptoms and at least 25% are unable to return to full duty.

REFERENCES

1. Freedman BJ. Dr Edward Wilson of the Antarctic; a biographical sketch, followed by an inquiry into the nature of his last illness. Proc R Soc Med 1954;47:183–9.
2. Horn CE. Acute ischaemia of the anterior tibial muscle and the long extensor muscles of the toes. J Bone Joint Surg Am 1945;27(4):615–22.
3. Leach RE, Hammond G, Stryker WS. Anterior tibial compartment syndrome. Acute and chronic. J Bone Joint Surg Am 1967;49(3):451–62.
4. Blandy J, Fuller R. March gangrene: ischaemic myositis of the leg muscle from exercise. J Bone Joint Surg Br 1957;39B(4):679–93.
5. Brennan FH, Kane SF. Diagnosis, treatment options, and rehabilitation of chronic lower leg exertional compartment syndrome. Curr Sports Med Rep 2003;2(5):247–50.
6. Fronek J, Mubarak SJ, Hargens AR, et al. Management of chronic exertional anterior compartment syndrome of the lower extremity. Clin Orthop Relat Res 1987;220:217–27.
7. Gill CS, Halstead ME, Matava MJ. Chronic exertional compartment syndrome of the leg in athletes: evaluation and management. Phys Sportsmed 2010;2(38):126–32.
8. Birtles DB, Rayson MP, Casey A, et al. Venous obstruction in healthy limbs: a model for chronic compartment syndrome? Med Sci Sports Exerc 2003;25(10):1638–44.

9. Edmundsson D, Toolanen G, Sojka P. Chronic compartment syndrome also affects non-athletic subjects: a prospective study of 63 cases with exercise-induced lower leg pain. Acta Orthop 2007;78(1):136–42.

10. Pedowitz RA, Hargens AR, Mubarak SJ, et al. Modified criteria for the objective diagnosis of chronic compartment syndrome of the leg. Am J Sports Med 1990; 18(1):35–40.

11. Qvarfordt P, Christenson JT, Eklöf B, et al. Intramuscular pressure, muscle blood flow, and skeletal muscle metabolism in chronic anterior tibial compartment syndrome. Clin Orthop Relat Res 1983;(179):284–90.

12. Styf JR, Korner LM. Chronic anterior-compartment syndrome of the leg. J Bone Joint Surg Am 1986;68(9):1338–47.

13. Waterman BR, Liu J, Newcomb R, et al. Risk factors for chronic exertional compartment syndrome in a physically active military population. Am J Sports Med 2013;41(11):2545–9.

14. Barnes M. Diagnosis and management of chronic compartment syndromes: a review of the literature. Br J Sports Med 1997;31(1):21–7.

15. Lee CH, Lee KH, Lee SH, et al. Chronic exertional compartment syndrome in adductor pollicis muscle: case report. J Hand Surg Am 2012;37A:2310.

16. Reid RL, Travis RT. Acute necrosis of the second interosseous compartment of the hand. J Bone Joint Surg Am 1973;55A:1095–7.

17. Harrison JW, Thomas P, Aster A, et al. Chronic exertional compartment syndrome of the forearm in elite rowers: a technique for mini-open fasciotomy and a report of six cases. Hand (N Y) 2013;8(4):450–3.

18. Tompkins DG. Exercise myopathy of the extensor carpi ulnaris muscle. Report of a case. J Bone Joint Surg Am 1977;59A:407–8.

19. Winkes MB, Luiten EJ, van Zoest WJ, et al. Long-term results of surgical decompression of chronic exertional compartment syndrome of the forearm in motocross racers. Am J Sports Med 2012;40(2):452–8.

20. Orava S, Rantanen J, Kujala UM. Fasciotomy of the posterior femoral muscle compartment in athletes. Int J Sports Med 1998;19(1):71–5.

21. Raether PM, Lutter LD. Recurrent compartment syndrome in the posterior thigh. Report of a case. Am J Sports Med 1982;10:40–3.

22. Mollica MB. Chronic exertional compartment syndrome of the foot. A case report. J Am Podiatr Med Assoc 1998;88(1):21–4.

23. Davis DE, Raikin S, Garras DN, et al. Characteristics of patients with chronic exertional compartment syndrome. Foot Ankle Int 2013;34(10):1349–54.

24. Touliopolous S, Hershman EB. Lower leg pain. Diagnosis and treatment of compartment syndromes and other pain syndromes of the leg. Sports Med 1999;27(3):193–204.

25. Waterman BR, Laughlin MD, Kilcoyne K, et al. Surgical treatment of chronic exertional compartment syndrome of the leg: failure rates and postoperative disability in an active patient population. J Bone Joint Surg Am 2013;95:592–6.

26. Detmer DE, Sharpe K, Sufit RL, et al. Chronic compartment syndrome: diagnosis, management, and outcomes. Am J Sports Med 1985;13(3):162–70.

27. Howard JL, Mohtadi NG, Wiley JP. Evaluation of outcomes in patients following surgical treatment of chronic exertional compartment syndrome in the leg. Clin J Sport Med 2000;10:176–84.

28. Pedowitz RA, Hargens AR. Acute and chronic compartment syndromes. In: Garrett EW, Speer KP, Kirkendall DT, editors. Principles and practice of orthopaedic sports medicine. Philadelphia: Lippincott, Williams, and Wilkins; 2001. p. 87–97.

29. Garcia-Mata S, Hidalgo-Ovejero A, Martinez-Grande M. Chronic exertional compartment syndrome of the legs in adolescents. J Pediatr Orthop 2001;21(3): 328–34.
30. Hurschler C, Vanderby R, Martinez DA, et al. Mechanical and biochemical analyses of tibial compartment fascia in chronic compartment syndrome. Ann Biomed Eng 1994;22(3):272–9.
31. Fraipont MJ, Adamson GJ. Chronic exertional compartment syndrome. J Am Acad Orthop Surg 2003;11(4):268–76.
32. Schissel DJ, Godwin J. Effort related chronic compartment syndrome of the lower extremity. Mil Med 1999;164:830–2.
33. Tubb CC, Vermillon D. Chronic exertional compartment syndrome after minor injury to the lower extremity. Mil Med 2001;166(4):366–8.
34. Rowdon GA, Richardson JK, Hoffmann P, et al. Chronic anterior compartment syndrome and deep peroneal nerve function. Clin J Sport Med 2001;11:229–33.
35. Winkes MB, Hooeveen AR, Houterman S, et al. Compartment pressure curves predict surgical outcome in chronic deep posterior compartment syndrome. Am J Sports Med 2012;40(4):1899–905.
36. Aweid O, Del Buono A, Malliaras P, et al. Systematic review and recommendations for intracompartmental pressure monitoring in diagnosing chronic exertional compartment syndrome of the leg. Clin J Sport Med 2012;22(4):356–70.
37. Lauder TD, Stuart MJ, Amrami KK, et al. Exertional compartment syndrome and the role of magnetic resonance imaging. Am J Phys Med Rehabil 2002;81(4):315–9.
38. Eskelin MK, Lotjonen JM, Mantysaari MJ. Chronic exertional compartment syndrome: MR imaging at 0.1T compared with tissue pressure measurement. Radiology 1998;206:333–7.
39. van den Brand JG, Verleisdonk EJ, van der Werken C. Near infrared spectroscopy in the diagnosis of chronic exertional compartment syndrome. Am J Sports Med 2004;32(2):452–6.
40. van den Brand JG, Nelson T, Verleisdonk EJ, et al. The diagnostic value of intracompartmental pressure measurement, magnetic resonance imaging, and near-infrared spectroscopy in chronic exertional compartment syndrome. A prospective study in 50 patients. Am J Sports Med 2005;33(5):699–704.
41. Packer JD, Day MS, Nguyen JT, et al. Functional outcomes and patient satisfaction after fasciotomy for chronic external compartment syndrome. Am J Sports Med 2013;40(4):430–6.
42. Blackman PG, Simmons LR, Crossley KM. Treatment of chronic exertional anterior compartment syndrome with massage: a pilot study. Clin J Sport Med 1998;8:14–7.
43. Beckham SG, Grana WA, Buckley P. A comparison of anterior compartment pressures in competitive runners and cyclists. Am J Sports Med 1993;21:36–40.
44. Diebal AR, Gregory R, Alitz C, et al. Forefoot running improves pain and disability associated with chronic exertional compartment syndrome. Am J Sports Med 2012;40(5):1060–7.
45. Slimmon D, Bennell K, Brukner P, et al. Long-term outcome of fasciotomy with partial fasciectomy for chronic exertional compartment syndrome of the lower leg. Am J Sports Med 2002;30(4):581–8.
46. Schepsis AA, Fitzgerald M, Nicoletta R. Revision surgery for exertional anterior compartment syndrome of the lower leg. Technique, findings, and results. Am J Sports Med 2005;33(7):1041–8.
47. Schepsis AA, Gill SS, Foster TA. Fasciotomy for exertional anterior compartment syndrome: is lateral compartment release necessary? Am J Sports Med 1999; 27(4):430–5.

48. Rollins DL, Bernhard VM, Towne JB. Fasciotomy: an appraisal of controversial issues. Arch Surg 1981;116(11):1474–81.
49. Ernst CB, Kaufer H. Fibulectomy-fasciotomy. An important adjunct in management of lower extremity arterial trauma. J Trauma 1971;11:365–80.
50. Maheshwari R, Taitsman LA, Barei DP. Single-incision fasciotomy for compartmental syndrome of the leg in patients with diaphyseal tibial fractures. J Orthop Trauma 2008;22(10):723–30.
51. Charles A, Rockwood J, editors. Rockwood & Green's fractures in adults, vol. 1, 4th edition. Philadelphia: Lippincott-Raven Publishers; 1996.
52. Mubarak SJ, Owen CA. Double-incision fasciotomy of the leg for decompression in compartment syndrome. J Bone Joint Surg Am 1977;59(2):184–7.
53. Rorabeck CH, Bourne RB, Fowler PJ. The surgical treatment of exertional compartment syndrome in athletes. J Bone Joint Surg Am 1983;65(5):1245–51.
54. Davey JR, Rorabeck CH, Fowler PJ. The tibialis posterior muscle comparmtnet. An unrecognized cause of exertional compartment syndrome. Am J Sports Med 1984;12(5):391–7.
55. Ruland RT, April EW, Meinhard BP. Tibialis posterior muscle: the fifth compartment? J Orthop Trauma 1992;6(3):347–51.
56. Hislop M, Tierney P, Murray P, et al. Chronic exertional compartment syndrome: the controversial "fifth" compartment of the leg. Am J Sports Med 2003;31(5):770–6.
57. Knight J, Daniels M, Robertson W. Endoscopic compartment release for chronic exertional compartment syndrome. Arthrosc Tech 2013;2(2):187–90.
58. Lohrer H, Nauck T. Endoscopically assisted release for exertional compartment syndromes of the lower leg. Arch Orthop Trauma Surg 2007;127:827–34.
59. Sebik A, Dogan A. A technique for arthroscopic fasciotomy for the chronic exertional tibialis anterior compartment syndrome. Knee Surg Sports Traumatol Arthrosc 2008;16(5):531–4.
60. Stein DA, Sennett BJ. One-portal endoscopically assisted fasciotomy for exertional compartment syndrome. Arthroscopy 2005;21(1):108–12.
61. Wittstein J, Moorman CT, Levin LS. Endoscopic compartment release for chronic exertional compartment syndrome: surgical technique and results. Am J Sports Med 2010;28:1661–6.
62. Flautt W, Miller J. Post-surgical rehabilitation following fasciotomies for bilateral chronic exertional compartment syndrome in a special forces soldier: a case report. Int J Sports Phys Ther 2013;8(5):701–15.
63. Schubert AG. Exertional compartment syndrome: review of the literature and proposed rehabilitation guidelines following surgical release. Int J Sports Phys Ther 2011;6(2):126–41.
64. Schepsis AA, Martini D, Corbett M. Surgical management of exertional compartment syndrome of the lower leg. Long-term followup. Am J Sports Med 1993;21(6):811–7.
65. Almdahl SM, Samdal F. Fasciotomy for chronic compartment syndrome. Acta Orthop Scand 1989;60(2):210–1.
66. Roberts AJ, Krishnasamy P, Quayle JM, et al. Outcomes of surgery for chronic exertional compartment syndrome in a military population. J R Army Med Corps 2014. http://dx.doi.org/10.1136/jramc-2013-000191. [Epub ahead of print]. PMID:24687656.

Shoulder Instability in the Military

Guillaume D. Dumont, MD[a],*, Petar Golijanin, BS[b], Matthew T. Provencher, MD[c]

KEYWORDS

- Shoulder dislocation • Glenohumeral instability • Bankart lesion • Glenoid bone loss
- ALPSA • HAGL • Labrum • Military

KEY POINTS

- An understanding of risk factors for recurrent instability is critical in selecting the appropriate treatment plan, including the most appropriate surgical procedure, for each patient. The duties of military personnel place them at high risk for shoulder instability.
- Advanced imaging modalities are useful in associated lesions in the unstable shoulder. Although MRI is useful for identifying associated labral or capsular injuries (ALPSA, HAGL, Bankart, GLAD, rotator cuff tear), CT is most effective for identifying and quantifying glenoid bone loss.
- The lateral decubitus position with gentle balanced suspension of the arm offers excellent visualization of the entire glenbohumeral joint, thus facilitating the treatment of isolocated or circumferential labral lesions.
- Bony reconstruction procedures, including coracoid transfer or distal tibial allograft, should be considered for patients with significant glenoid bone loss, or patients who have recurrent instability after soft tissue reconstruction.

INTRODUCTION

The geometry of the glenohumeral joint allows for a large arc of motion, but also places the joint at higher risk for instability. The incidence of glenohumeral instability in the military has been estimated to be 1.69 per 1000 person-years (compared with 0.08 per 1000 person-years for the general US population).[1] Male gender, age younger than 30, service in the army, and junior enlisted rank have been found to be significant demographic risk factors associated with instability.[1] The unique job characteristics and duties of military personnel predispose them to initial instability events, and also recurrent instability before or after surgery.

[a] Department of Orthopaedic Surgery and Sports Medicine, University of South Carolina School of Medicine, 2 Medical Park, Suite 404, Columbia, SC 29203, USA; [b] Sports Medicine Service, Massachusetts General Hospital, 175 Cambridge Street, Suite 400, Boston, MA 02114, USA; [c] Sports Medicine Service, Harvard Medical School, Massachusetts General Hospital, 175 Cambridge Street, Suite 400, Boston, MA 02114, USA
* Corresponding author.
E-mail address: gddumont@gmail.com

Clin Sports Med 33 (2014) 707–720
http://dx.doi.org/10.1016/j.csm.2014.06.006
0278-5919/14/$ – see front matter © 2014 Elsevier Inc. All rights reserved.

Male gender is predominant in reported series of patients with shoulder instability, including those in the military population. Owens and colleagues[2] studied the epidemiology of shoulder instability at the US Military Academy and found similar 1-year incidence proportions in each gender (2.9% in males and 2.5% in females). A total of 84.6% of the instability events were subluxations and 15.4% were dislocations. A total of 80.3% of instability events were anterior, 12.3% were posterior, and 9.4% were multidirectional. Injuries in their series were approximately evenly divided between contact and noncontact injuries. Other than sporting activities, military-specific activities, such as the military movement gymnastics course, the indoor obstacle course test, the army physical fitness test, and military training, were cited as common injury mechanisms.

Patients with anterior shoulder dislocation events at age younger than 20 have a 90% rate of recurrence, whereas patients older than 40 years have only a 10% recurrence rate but are more prone to rotator cuff injuries.[3] A study of 3854 military personal showed that with every 1-year increase in age, there was a 7% decrease in the likelihood of recurrent instability after Bankart repair. Patients that compete in high-level and contact sports are also at an increased risk of recurrence if treated nonoperatively. The duties of military personnel place them in the same subset as high-level contact athletes for risk assessment.[4]

Although glenohumeral dislocations have received significant attention in the literature, subluxations have a high incidence in the young athlete. A series of 27 military patients sustaining a first-time subluxation revealed a Bankart lesion in 26 of 27 patients, and Hill-Sachs lesion in 25 of 27 patients (on preoperative magnetic resonance imaging [MRI]). Thirteen of 14 of these patients who underwent surgery had a Bankart lesion noted intraoperatively. Four of 13 patients that did not have surgery had recurrent instability.[5] Subluxation events are capable of causing significant anatomic lesions, and should not be dismissed despite their less dramatic presentation than dislocations.

PATIENT EVALUATION

A directed history and physical examination of the shoulder can elucidate much information about the injury pattern of the shoulder. Mechanism of injury and position of the shoulder during dislocation is important. Posterior directed force to the arm while the shoulder is abducted and externally rotated is characteristic of anterior instability. Pain with axial load to a forward flexed arm should raise suspicion for posterior instability.[6]

Physical examination should include thorough inspection and range of motion evaluation. Provocative maneuvers include the apprehension test/relocation sign, anterior and posterior load and shift test, jerk test, and Kim test. The apprehension test and relocation sign are the most common clinical finding in patients with anterior instability.[7] The jerk test is more sensitive for identification of predominantly posterior labral lesions, whereas the Kim test is more sensitive for identification of posteroinferior labral lesions.[8]

Boileau and colleagues[9] found that anterior shoulder hyperlaxity, inferior shoulder hyperlaxity, glenoid bone loss, and the presence of a Hill-Sachs lesion increase the risk of postoperative recurrence of instability. It is important to identify these factors in patients presenting with shoulder instability. Anterior shoulder laxity can be defined as external rotation of greater than 90 degrees with the arm at the side. This is usually seen bilaterally and associated with general ligamentous laxity. Inferior shoulder laxity can be defined as difference of 20 degrees or greater on hyperabduction of the shoulder (Gagey test). Those with greater than 90 degrees external rotation with the arm at the side, and/or a positive Gagey test have increased recurrence risk after instability repair.

On initial presentation of a patient with traumatic shoulder dislocation, true antero-posterior, axillary lateral, and scapular Y views should be obtained. In patients with a history of recurrent anterior instability, further imaging views can be obtained, including the Stryker notch, the apical oblique, Didiee, or West Point views.[10,11] As described later, axial imaging, such as MRI or computed tomography (CT), is often necessary to identify associated lesions that may affect prognosis and treatment selection.

ASSOCIATED LESIONS OF SHOULDER INSTABILITY

Certain bony and soft tissue lesions associated with shoulder instability increase the risk of recurrent instability in patients treated nonoperatively, or can increase the risk of failure after surgical treatment. A high degree of clinical suspicion is required in identifying these lesions, preferably in the preoperative setting using appropriate imaging techniques. The most commonly identified lesions are detachment of the inferior glenohumeral ligament (IGHL), Bankart lesion, bony Bankart, Hill-Sachs lesion, humeral avulsion of the glenohumeral ligament (HAGL), anterior labral periosteal sleeve avulsion (ALSPA), and glenolabral articular disruption (GLAD). Glenoid bone loss is commonly associated with cases of recurrent instability. Its presence should be recognized to avoid failed surgical treatment. These anatomic lesions are discussed in further detail next.

Ligaments contributing to glenohumeral stability include the superior glenohumeral ligament, middle glenohumeral ligament, and IGHL. The IGHL is the primary restraint to anterior translation of the humeral head when the shoulder is abducted to 90 degrees and externally rotated, the typical position of instability. Recurrent episodes of instability further damage and stretch this ligamentous structure. In a cadaveric study, sectioning of the IGHL at the level of the anteroinferior glenoid resulted in only slight increases in anterior translation, thus a stretching or elongation of the capsular tissue or IGHL is likely necessary to produce anterior glenohumeral instability.[12]

Bankart Lesion

The Bankart lesion (detachment of the anteroinferior labrum) has been reported in up to 90% of traumatic anterior shoulder dislocations.[5] The lesion is well seen on MRI (**Fig. 1**). In an arthroscopic evaluation of patients with shoulder instability, Hintermann and Gachter[13] noted that 87% of patients with shoulder instability had anterior labral tears, and 79% had anterior capsular insufficiency.

Bony Bankart/Glenoid bone loss

A fracture of the anteroinferior glenoid is referred to as a bony Bankart lesion. Recurrent instability can cause erosive or attritional loss of the glenoid rim causing progressive instability. Loss of greater than 20% of the glenoid rim has been shown to cause significant recurrent instability and usually requires surgical correction of the bony deficiency.[14] This number is not absolute and other factors may contribute to failure at even lesser amounts of glenoid bone loss. This deficiency may be suggested by a break in the sclerotic line encircling the glenoid rim on the anteroposterior view of the shoulder. Axillary views of shoulder, such as the Bernageau view, can also show a break in the sclerotic line of the anterior glenoid rim.[15]

Glenoid bone loss is a substantial contributing factor to recurrent instability and failure after surgical repair of unstable shoulder.[16,17] Burkhart and De Beer[18] reported a recurrence rate after arthroscopic Bankart repair of 4% in patients without significant bony defects and 67% in patients with significant bony defects. Contact athletes had recurrence rates of 6.5% in those without significant bony defects and 89% in those

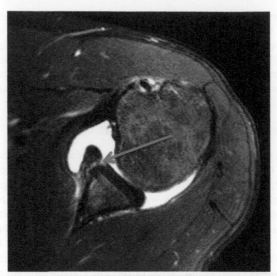

Fig. 1. MRI arthrogram showing a detached anteroinferior labrum (*arrow*; the Bankart lesion).

with significant bony defects. Although military personnel were not specifically studied, the contact athlete and solider in many ways participate in similar high-risk activities involving the shoulder. Itoi and colleagues[14] in a cadaveric study found that shoulders with 21% or greater of the anterior glenoid width missing were at risk for recurrent instability and loss of range of motion after Bankart repair. They postulate that the loss of range of motion stems from the need to pretension the capsule to close the gap between it and the diminished glenoid rim.

Imaging modalities for measurement of bone loss

Despite the possibility of quantifying glenoid bone loss arthroscopically, preoperative recognition of glenoid bone loss is critical, and helps the surgeon select the appropriate surgical procedure. Imaging and measurement techniques best suited for accurate assessment of bone loss have been a popular topic of investigation. Although radiographs and MRI can be used, three-dimensional CT is the most reliable modality for quantifying bone loss.[19,20] Some authors have advocated the use of bilateral CT scans, which allows the comparison of the injured glenoid with the contralateral glenoid. The patient does not incur additional radiation if images of the contralateral shoulder are obtained during the same scan.

Various measurement techniques have been described. Most techniques are easily and reliably performed by first obtaining a three-dimensional reconstruction of the CT scan, and manipulating the scan to obtain an en face view of the glenoid. **Fig. 2** shows the en face view of the glenoid on a three-dimensional reconstruction of a CT of the shoulder. A best-fit circle is then created over the inferior aspect of the glenoid.[17,21] In a normal glenoid, the best-fit circle over the inferior glenoid is completely filled with bone. In cases of anterior glenoid bone loss, the width of missing bone along the line of the circle's diameter is divided by the diameter of the circle, and represents the percent bone loss.[22] The same concept can be applied using the area of the circle as opposed to a one-dimensional measurement of its width, the area of the circle where bone is missing divided by the total surface area of the circle represents a

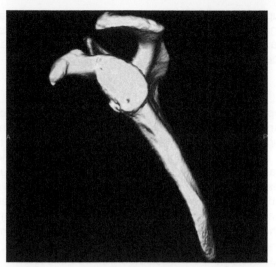

Fig. 2. The "en face" view on a three-dimensional reconstruction of a CT of the shoulder.

two-dimensional percentage of glenoid bone loss. Methods to measure bone loss two dimensionally have been described that require specialized software or calculations based on mathematical formulas of circle geometry.[23,24] The glenoid arc angle method proposes measuring one angle, from the superior intersection of the glenoid defect and the best-fit circle, to the center of the circle, to the inferior intersection of the glenoid defect and the best-fit circle. This angle directly correlates to the percent bone loss, thus knowing the threshold "glenoid arc angle" could be beneficial in guiding the clinician when deciding between soft tissue or bony reconstruction.[25,26] Gerber and Nyffeler[27] mention that according to biomechanical evaluations, if the superoinferior extension of the glenoid rim lesion is larger than half the maximal diameter of the circle, a resultant 30% loss of resistance to dislocation is seen. Although the information is useful in understanding the biomechanics of the glenohumeral joint, this technique does not provide a method of numerically quantifying glenoid bone loss.

Regardless of which method is used, it is important not to use one- or two-dimensional measurements interchangeably, because the values obtained do not represent the same amount of bone loss. A certain percent area of bone loss is equivalent to a smaller percentage of the width of the circle.

Arthroscopic quantification of bone loss
The degree of glenoid and humeral head bone loss should ideally be identified preoperatively, because this allows decision making in the clinic setting with the patient based on a shared decision-making model. However, arthroscopic quantification of bone loss has been described using a glenoid "bare spot," which serves to mark the mid point of the glenoid. This landmark can be used to measure the length of bone anterior and posterior to it, and thus calculate the percent missing bone.[28] The reliability of the bare spot as a consistent landmark has been questioned.[29,30] Detterline and colleagues[31] described the secant chord theory to measure bone loss during arthroscopy. The method was shown to be more accurate than the glenoid bare spot method, but requires additional mathematical calculations. The inverted pear glenoid has been described as a glenoid with its inferior aspect having a smaller

width than the superior aspect (the inverse of the normal anatomic appearance). The inverted pear glenoid represents bone loss of at least 25%.[32] Patients with this degree of bone loss are at high risk of failure after arthroscopic Bankart repair, and bony procedures should be considered.[22,33]

ALPSA Lesion

ALPSA lesions represent an avulsion of the labrum and anterior glenoid/scapular periosteum. These structures displace medially and rotate inferiorly on the scapular neck, eventually healing in this position, leading to incompetence of the labrum/IGHL (**Fig. 3**).[34] When compared with patients with Bankart lesions, those with ALPSA lesions showed a higher number of preoperative dislocations, larger Hill-Sachs lesions, and increased likelihood of an engaging Hill-Sachs lesion. In addition the rate of recurrent instability after surgery is increased.[35,36] Care must be taken if performing a Bankart repair in patients with this lesion to properly elevate the soft tissue sleeve to the extent that the subscapularis muscle belly can be visualized medially. Alternatively, bony reconstruction procedures should often be considered, given that these patients may also have significant associated glenoid bone loss.

Hill-Sachs Lesion

The Hill-Sachs lesion is a compression fracture of the posterosuperolateral humeral head that is coupled with anterior shoulder instability events.[37] It was first described by Hill and Sachs as a groove defect of the humeral head caused during anterior dislocation, and is extremely common after anterior instability events.[37,38] Most lesions are visible on radiograph. MRI has been very effective in determining the size and location of these lesions, with 91% sensitivity and 97% specificity.[39] The lesions can also easily be seen on CT (**Fig. 4**). When treating a patient with both glenoid and humeral bone deficiency it is important to consider their relationship. Yamamoto and colleagues[40] introduced the glenoid track concept in cadaver study to help predict whether a Hill-Sachs lesion will engage the anterior glenoid.[37]

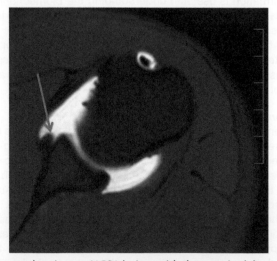

Fig. 3. MRI arthrogram showing an ALPSA lesion, with the anterior labrum (*arrow*) and periosteal tissue avulsed and scarred to the medial glenoid neck.

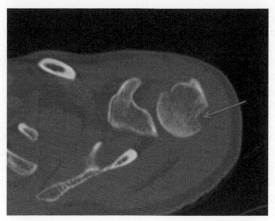

Fig. 4. Axial cut of a shoulder CT showing a large Hill-Sachs lesion (*arrow*).

HAGL

HAGL lesion is an avulsion of the IGHL from its humeral attachment.[41] It is less commonly identified than the Bankart lesion after instability episodes, but similarly results in insufficiency of the IGHL. Although intraoperative diagnosis of these lesions is possible when examining the inferior aspect of the glenohumeral joint, preoperative identification is ideal. MRI arthrogram can be helpful in identifying the HAGL lesion, and shows pooling of the contrast material in the now incompetent axillary recess (**Fig. 5**).[42] HAGL lesions are most often associated with anterior avulsion of IGHL, but can be associated with posterior avulsion.[42] Humeral reattachment of the IGHL can be performed arthroscopically but some authors suggest that an open approach results in better outcomes.[42]

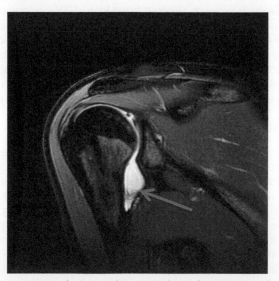

Fig. 5. Coronal view on MRI arthrogram shows pooling of contrast material adjacent to the proximal medial humeral shaft (*arrow*), representing a HAGL lesion.

GLAD Lesion

GLAD lesion represents injury to the anterior glenoid cartilage, usually in the setting of an anterior labral tear. It is important to recognize it because it can be a source of persistent anterior shoulder pain. The injury may range from a cartilaginous flap to a depressed osteochondral injury of the anterior glenoid.[43]

TREATMENT
Initial Treatment

The mainstay of treatment of the dislocated shoulder has traditionally been the use of a sling for comfort until initial symptoms subside, followed by progressive mobilization and strengthening. No advantage has been observed with prolonged immobilization.[44–46] Immobilization with the arm externally rotated has been proposed, with the rationale being that in external rotation, the displaced anterior capsulolabral structures are reduced back and compressed to their origin on the anterior glenoid where they can heal.[47–49] Although promising results were noted in an initial study of this technique, these findings have not been replicated in subsequent series.[44,47,50–52] Our current strategy for initial treatment of the dislocated shoulder remains brief immobilization for comfort, followed by progressive mobilization, and a discussion of risks and benefits of surgical stabilization versus nonoperative care.

Surgical Treatment

There is increasing evidence that surgical treatment of first time dislocators may be indicated.[53–55] Recurrence rates in patients treated nonsurgically has been reported between 60% and 90%.[56] The military population presents a distinct group of individuals who typically have several factors that place them at higher risk for recurrence, including young age, high level of physical activity, and a large predominance of male patients.

Surgical treatment of anterior instability typically falls into two categories: soft tissue or bony reconstructions. The choice of surgical procedure should be influenced by the severity of associated lesions discussed previously. Glenoid bone loss exerts the most influence in our decision process. Glenoid bone loss of 20% or greater should lead to consideration of bony reconstruction procedures. In the setting of associated lesions, such as HAGL or ALPSA lesions, patients with lesser degrees of bone loss may also benefit from bony reconstruction.[18,57] Preoperative risk factors can be used to calculate an Instability Severity Index Score to help guide surgeons in selecting between arthroscopic Bankart repair and bony reconstruction options, such as the Bristow-Latarjet procedure, iliac crest bone graft, or osteochondral allograft reconstruction.[58]

ARTHROSCOPIC SURGICAL MANAGEMENT

Military personal with shoulder instability have been successfully treated using open and arthroscopic treatment methods.[59] Although open Bankart repair has been considered the gold standard for management of anterior shoulder instability, clinical outcomes show no difference between open or arthroscopic Bankart repair.[60,61] A meta-analysis of patients treated with capsulolabral repair using suture anchors (234 arthroscopic and 267 open) found similar rates of recurrent instability (6% vs 6.7%) and need for reoperation (4.7% and 6.6%).[62] Another systematic review 1781 patients from 26 studies showed no statistically significant difference in rates of recurrent instability after arthroscopic or open Bankart repair (11% vs 8%, respectively).[63] Waterman and colleagues[4] report a series of 3854 US Army patients that underwent arthroscopic or open Bankart repair. At 2 to 7 years follow-up, 5% of patients had undergone revision surgery and 8.8% were medically discharged with complaints of shoulder instability, thus amounting to a combined failure rate of 13.8%. Their patients were predominantly men (92%) with a mean age of 28 years. These factors may account for a recurrence rate slightly higher than otherwise reported in civilian populations. Their study showed higher failure rates after open repair compared with arthroscopic repair (17.9% vs 13.0%). Arthroscopic technique has become the overwhelmingly popular treatment choice for cases that can be treated with soft tissue repair only.

Patient Set Up and Preoperative Considerations

Regional anesthesia supplemented with light general anesthesia allows for optimal pain control postoperatively. The procedure can be performed with the patient in the beach-chair position or lateral decubitus position, although the authors exclusively use the lateral decubitus position. The beach-chair position provides the ability to visualize the anterosuperior, anterior, and inferior aspects of the glenohumeral joint, and ease of conversion to open procedures if necessary. The lateral decubitus position with gentle balanced suspension is the senior author's preferred position for instability repairs. It provides excellent visualization of the entire capsulolabral complex and provides greater visibility and ease of access of the entire glenohumeral joint, improved ability to manipulate instruments, and to make adequate passes through soft tissue for optimal repair.[64] Before the procedure, a thorough examination under anesthesia including the load shift test can help clarify the patient's pathology with regards to the extent and direction of instability.

Surgical Technique

Diagnostic arthroscopy confirms the expected pathology, and can identify additional lesions in the shoulder. After initial arthroscopy through the posterior portal, visualization through an anterosuperior portal is useful to appreciate the full extent of pathology to the capsulolabral tissue and the degree of glenoid bone loss. Visualization through this portal also provides a complete appreciation of lesions extending to the posterior labrum. We prefer the lateral decubitus position with balanced suspension in part because of the excellent ability it provides to visualize the entire 360 degrees of the glenoid labrum.

After identification of the area of injury, the scarred capsulolabral tissue is elevated off of the glenoid. Anteriorly, visualization of the posterior subscapularis muscle indicates adequate dissection medially, which allows appropriate mobilization of the tissues back to their origin. The capsulolabral tissue should float up to the glenoid face after adequate mobilization. The glenoid rim and scapular neck are prepared with a rasp and arthroscopic shaver to expose a bleeding bed of bone. Typical anteroinferior tears require at least three anchors between the 6- and 3-o'clock positions on the glenoid face. More anchors are used as needed for tears extending posteriorly or involving the superior labrum. Sutures are passed through the capsular tissues using a curved suture-passing device, and should penetrate tissues inferior to the level of anchor, thus shifting the tissue superiorly when the sutures are tied. Sutures should be tied in such a fashion to avoid bulky knots that could abrade the humeral head articular cartilage, or knotless anchors can alternatively be used.

Surgical Treatment of Significant Bone Loss

The Bristow-Latarjet procedure involves transfer of the coracoid and the attached conjoint tendon (short head of the biceps and coracobrachialis) through a split in the subscapularis tendon, to the anterior scapular neck at the anterior glenoid rim.[65,66] The bony surface area of the anterior glenoid is increased, but more importantly a soft tissue sling effect is created by the inferior portion of the subscapularis tendon, which is compressed posteriorly by the conjoint tendon with abduction and external rotation of the shoulder. Although most commonly performed through an open deltopectoral approach, the Latarjet procedure has also been described using arthroscopic technique.[67] Bhatia and colleagues[68] performed a systematic review of outcomes after the Latarjet procedure. Eight studies reported recurrence rates of 0% to 8% with follow-up ranging between 6 months and 14 years. Schroder and colleagues[69] examined long-term recurrent instability rates for the modified Bristow procedure in Naval Academy midshipmen. A rate of 15.4% recurrent instability (9.6% dislocation, 5.8% subluxation) was noted in this series of 52 shoulders in 49 patients with a mean follow-up of 26 years.

Revision situations, where a coracoid graft may no longer be available, may require the use of autograft iliac crest augmentation. Osteochondral allograft transfer from the tibial plafond has been described, with the geometry of the tibial plafond bearing resemblance to that of the glenoid.[70–72] These techniques do not offer the benefits of the soft tissue sling provided by the subscapularis and conjoint tendon after Bristow-Latarjet reconstruction, but may be optimal to reconstruct the glenoid in cases of severe bone loss.

Postoperative Care

Rehabilitation protocols should be emphasized to the patient preoperatively, so that a clear understanding exists of postoperative limitations and of the time required before return to activities. Most repairs are immobilized following the procedure, with anterior repairs placed in an abduction sling. Posterior repairs are placed in an external rotation sling to avoid stress to the posterior capsular tissues. Physical therapy begins 7 to 10 days after surgery, with passive and active assisted motion for the initial 4 weeks after surgery. Limitations on motion in this early phase are placed at 130 degrees of forward flexion and 30 degrees of external rotation, and can be progressed gradually to full range of motion afterward. Active range of motion is added to the regimen at 6 to 8 weeks after surgery, followed by resistive strengthening at 8 to 12 weeks. Full return to sports and activities is typically expected at 4 to 6 months after surgery.[64]

SUMMARY

Shoulder instability is common in military populations, and this demographic represents individuals at high risk for recurrence. Surgical management is often indicated, especially in high-demand young individuals, and provides a predictable return to military duties. Accurate recognition of glenoid bone loss and other associated anatomic lesions is of importance for appropriate selection between arthroscopic capsulolabral repair and bony reconstruction procedures. A thorough understanding of underlying pathology, diagnostic testing, and available treatment options provides for optimal care of the unstable shoulder.

REFERENCES

1. Owens BD, Dawson L, Burks R, et al. Incidence of shoulder dislocation in the United States military: demographic considerations from a high-risk population. J Bone Joint Surg Am 2009;91(4):791–6.
2. Owens BD, Duffey ML, Nelson BJ, et al. The incidence and characteristics of shoulder instability at the United States Military Academy. Am J Sports Med 2007;35(7):1168–73.

3. Mc LH, Cavallaro WU. Primary anterior dislocation of the shoulder. Am J Surg 1950;80(6):615–21 passim.
4. Waterman BR, Burns TC, McCriskin B, et al. Outcomes after Bankart repair in a military population: predictors for surgical revision and long-term disability. Arthroscopy 2014;30(2):172–7.
5. Owens BD, Nelson BJ, Duffey ML, et al. Pathoanatomy of first-time, traumatic, anterior glenohumeral subluxation events. J Bone Joint Surg Am 2010;92(7): 1605–11.
6. Dumont GD, Russell RD, Robertson WJ. Anterior shoulder instability: a review of pathoanatomy, diagnosis and treatment. Curr Rev Musculoskelet Med 2011; 4(4):200–7.
7. Lo IK, Nonweiler B, Woolfrey M, et al. An evaluation of the apprehension, relocation, and surprise tests for anterior shoulder instability. Am J Sports Med 2004;32(2):301–7.
8. Kim SH, Park JS, Jeong WK, et al. The Kim test: a novel test for posteroinferior labral lesion of the shoulder. A comparison to the jerk test. Am J Sports Med 2005;33(8):1188–92.
9. Boileau P, Villalba M, Héry JK, et al. Risk factors for recurrence of shoulder instability after arthroscopic Bankart repair. J Bone Joint Surg Am 2006;88(8):1755–63.
10. Pavlov H, Warren RF, Weiss CB Jr, et al. The roentgenographic evaluation of anterior shoulder instability. Clin Orthop Relat Res 1985;(194):153–8.
11. Rokous JR, Feagin JA, Abbott HG. Modified axillary roentgenogram. A useful adjunct in the diagnosis of recurrent instability of the shoulder. Clin Orthop Relat Res 1972;82:84–6.
12. Speer KP, Deng X, Borrero S, et al. Biomechanical evaluation of a simulated Bankart lesion. J Bone Joint Surg Am 1994;76(12):1819–26.
13. Hintermann B, Gachter A. Arthroscopic findings after shoulder dislocation. Am J Sports Med 1995;23(5):545–51.
14. Itoi E, Lee SB, Berglund LJ, et al. The effect of a glenoid defect on anteroinferior stability of the shoulder after Bankart repair: a cadaveric study. J Bone Joint Surg Am 2000;82(1):35–46.
15. Pansard E, Klouche S, Billot N, et al. Reliability and validity assessment of a glenoid bone loss measurement using the Bernageau profile view in chronic anterior shoulder instability. J Shoulder Elbow Surg 2013;22(9):1193–8.
16. Bollier MJ, Arciero R. Management of glenoid and humeral bone loss. Sports Med Arthrosc 2010;18(3):140–8.
17. Sugaya H, Moriishi J, Dohi M, et al. Glenoid rim morphology in recurrent anterior glenohumeral instability. J Bone Joint Surg Am 2003;85-A(5):878–84.
18. Burkhart SS, De Beer JF. Traumatic glenohumeral bone defects and their relationship to failure of arthroscopic Bankart repairs: significance of the inverted-pear glenoid and the humeral engaging Hill-Sachs lesion. Arthroscopy 2000; 16(7):677–94.
19. Auffarth A, Mayer M, Kofler B, et al. The interobserver reliability in diagnosing osseous lesions after first-time anterior shoulder dislocation comparing plain radiographs with computed tomography scans. J Shoulder Elbow Surg 2013; 22(11):1507–13.
20. Bishop JY, Jones GL, Rerko MA, et al. 3-D CT is the most reliable imaging modality when quantifying glenoid bone loss. Clin Orthop Relat Res 2013;471(4): 1251–6.
21. Huysmans PE, Haen PS, Kidd M, et al. The shape of the inferior part of the glenoid: a cadaveric study. J Shoulder Elbow Surg 2006;15(6):759–63.

22. Piasecki DP, Verma NN, Romeo AA, et al. Glenoid bone deficiency in recurrent anterior shoulder instability: diagnosis and management. J Am Acad Orthop Surg 2009;17(8):482–93.

23. Barchilon VS, Kotz E, Barchilon Ben-AV-M, et al. A simple method for quantitative evaluation of the missing area of the anterior glenoid in anterior instability of the glenohumeral joint. Skeletal Radiol 2008;37(8):731–6.

24. Magarelli N, Milano G, Sergio P, et al. Intra-observer and interobserver reliability of the "Pico" computed tomography method for quantification of glenoid bone defect in anterior shoulder instability. Skeletal Radiol 2009;38(11):1071–5.

25. Dumont GD, Russell RD, Browne MG, et al. Area-based determination of bone loss using the glenoid arc angle. Arthroscopy 2012;28(7):1030–5.

26. Nofsinger C, Browning B, Burkhart SS, et al. Objective preoperative measurement of anterior glenoid bone loss: a pilot study of a computer-based method using unilateral 3-dimensional computed tomography. Arthroscopy 2011;27(3):322–9.

27. Gerber C, Nyffeler RW. Classification of glenohumeral joint instability. Clin Orthop Relat Res 2002;(400):65–76.

28. Burkhart SS, Debeer JF, Tehrany AM, et al. Quantifying glenoid bone loss arthroscopically in shoulder instability. Arthroscopy 2002;18(5):488–91.

29. Saintmard B, Lecouvet F, Rubini A, et al. Is the bare spot a valid landmark for glenoid evaluation in arthroscopic Bankart surgery? Acta Orthop Belg 2009;75(6):736–42.

30. Kralinger F, Aigner F, Longato S, et al. Is the bare spot a consistent landmark for shoulder arthroscopy? A study of 20 embalmed glenoids with 3-dimensional computed tomographic reconstruction. Arthroscopy 2006;22(4):428–32.

31. Detterline AJ, Provencher MT, Ghodadra N, et al. A new arthroscopic technique to determine anterior-inferior glenoid bone loss: validation of the secant chord theory in a cadaveric model. Arthroscopy 2009;25(11):1249–56.

32. Lo IK, Parten PM, Burkhart SS. The inverted pear glenoid: an indicator of significant glenoid bone loss. Arthroscopy 2004;20(2):169–74.

33. Provencher MT, Bhatia S, Ghodadra NS, et al. Recurrent shoulder instability: current concepts for evaluation and management of glenoid bone loss. J Bone Joint Surg Am 2010;92(Suppl 2):133–51.

34. Neviaser TJ. The anterior labroligamentous periosteal sleeve avulsion lesion: a cause of anterior instability of the shoulder. Arthroscopy 1993;9(1):17–21.

35. Lee BG, Cho NS, Rhee YG. Anterior labroligamentous periosteal sleeve avulsion lesion in arthroscopic capsulolabral repair for anterior shoulder instability. Knee Surg Sports Traumatol Arthrosc 2011;19(9):1563–9.

36. Ozbaydar M, Elhassan B, Diller D, et al. Results of arthroscopic capsulolabral repair: Bankart lesion versus anterior labroligamentous periosteal sleeve avulsion lesion. Arthroscopy 2008;24(11):1277–83.

37. Metzger PD, Barlow B, Leonardelli D, et al. Clinical application of the "Glenoid Track" concept for defining humeral head engagement in anterior shoulder instability a preliminary report. Orthop J Sports Med 2013.

38. Hill HA, Sachs MD. The groove defect of the humeral head. A frequently unrecognized complication of dislocations of the shoulder joint. Radiology 1940;35:690–700.

39. Workman TL, Burkhard TK, Resnick D, et al. Hill-Sachs lesion: comparison of detection with MR imaging, radiography, and arthroscopy. Radiology 1992;185(3):847–52.

40. Yamamoto N, Itoi E, Abe H, et al. Contact between the glenoid and the humeral head in abduction, external rotation, and horizontal extension: a new concept of glenoid track. J Shoulder Elbow Surg 2007;16(5):649–56.

41. Wolf EM, Cheng JC, Dickson K. Humeral avulsion of glenohumeral ligaments as a cause of anterior shoulder instability. Arthroscopy 1995;11(5):600–7.
42. George MS, Khazzam M, Kuhn JE. Humeral avulsion of glenohumeral ligaments. J Am Acad Orthop Surg 2011;19(3):127–33.
43. Sanders TG, Tirman PF, Linares R, et al. The glenolabral articular disruption lesion: MR arthrography with arthroscopic correlation. AJR Am J Roentgenol 1999;172(1):171–5.
44. Paterson WH, Throckmrton TW, Koester M, et al. Position and duration of immobilization after primary anterior shoulder dislocation: a systematic review and meta-analysis of the literature. J Bone Joint Surg Am 2010;92(18):2924–33.
45. Pollock RG, Bigliani LU. Glenohumeral instability: evaluation and treatment. J Am Acad Orthop Surg 1993;1(1):24–32.
46. Hovelius L, Eriksson K, Fredin H, et al. Recurrences after initial dislocation of the shoulder. Results of a prospective study of treatment. J Bone Joint Surg Am 1983;65(3):343–9.
47. Itoi E, Hatakeyama Y, Kido T, et al. A new method of immobilization after traumatic anterior dislocation of the shoulder: a preliminary study. J Shoulder Elbow Surg 2003;12(5):413–5.
48. Scheibel M, Kkuke A, Nikulka C, et al. How long should acute anterior dislocations of the shoulder be immobilized in external rotation? Am J Sports Med 2009; 37(7):1309–16.
49. Siegler J, Proust J, Marcheiz PS, et al. Is external rotation the correct immobilisation for acute shoulder dislocation? An MRI study. Orthop Traumatol Surg Res 2010;96(4):329–33.
50. Itoi E, Hatakeyama Y, Sato T, et al. Immobilization in external rotation after shoulder dislocation reduces the risk of recurrence. A randomized controlled trial. J Bone Joint Surg Am 2007;89(10):2124–31.
51. Tanaka Y, Okamura K, Imai T. Effectiveness of external rotation immobilization in highly active young men with traumatic primary anterior shoulder dislocation or subluxation. Orthopedics 2010;33(9):670.
52. Finestone A, Milgrom C, Radeva-Petrova DR, et al. Bracing in external rotation for traumatic anterior dislocation of the shoulder. J Bone Joint Surg Br 2009; 91(7):918–21.
53. Bottoni CR, Wikkens JH, DeBerardino TM, et al. A prospective, randomized evaluation of arthroscopic stabilization versus nonoperative treatment in patients with acute, traumatic, first-time shoulder dislocations. Am J Sports Med 2002;30(4):576–80.
54. Law BK, Yung PS, Ho EP, et al. The surgical outcome of immediate arthroscopic Bankart repair for first time anterior shoulder dislocation in young active patients. Knee Surg Sports Traumatol Arthrosc 2008;16(2):188–93.
55. Boone JL, Arciero RA. First-time anterior shoulder dislocations: has the standard changed? Br J Sports Med 2010;44(5):355–60.
56. Marans HJ, Angel KR, Schemitsch EH, et al. The fate of traumatic anterior dislocation of the shoulder in children. J Bone Joint Surg Am 1992;74(8): 1242–4.
57. Porcellini G, Campi F, Pegreffie F, et al. Predisposing factors for recurrent shoulder dislocation after arthroscopic treatment. J Bone Joint Surg Am 2009;91(11): 2537–42.
58. Balg F, Boileau P. The instability severity index score. A simple pre-operative score to select patients for arthroscopic or open shoulder stabilisation. J Bone Joint Surg Br 2007;89(11):1470–7.

59. Middleton S, Guyver P, Boyd M, et al. Patient reported outcome measures in military patients with shoulder instability. J R Army Med Corps 2013;159(4):271–3.
60. Brophy RH, Marx RG. The treatment of traumatic anterior instability of the shoulder: nonoperative and surgical treatment. Arthroscopy 2009;25(3):298–304.
61. Pulavarti RS, Symes TH, Rangan A. Surgical interventions for anterior shoulder instability in adults. Cochrane Database Syst Rev 2009;(4):CD005077.
62. Petrera M, Patella V, Patella S, et al. A meta-analysis of open versus arthroscopic Bankart repair using suture anchors. Knee Surg Sports Traumatol Arthrosc 2010;18(12):1742–7.
63. Harris JD, Gupta AK, Mall NA, et al. Long-term outcomes after Bankart shoulder stabilization. Arthroscopy 2013;29(5):920–33.
64. Provencher MT, Ghodadra N, Romeo AA. Arthroscopic management of anterior instability: pearls, pitfalls, and lessons learned. Orthop Clin North Am 2010; 41(3):325–37.
65. Helfet AJ. Coracoid transplantation for recurring dislocation of the shoulder. J Bone Joint Surg Br 1958;40-B(2):198–202.
66. Latarjet M. Technic of coracoid preglenoid arthroereisis in the treatment of recurrent dislocation of the shoulder. Lyon Chir 1958;54(4):604–7 [in French].
67. Lafosse L, Boyle S. Arthroscopic Latarjet procedure. J Shoulder Elbow Surg 2010;19(2 Suppl):2–12.
68. Bhatia S, Frank RM, Ghodadra NS, et al. The outcomes and surgical techniques of the Latarjet procedure. Arthroscopy 2014;30(2):227–35.
69. Schroder DT, Provencher MT, Mologne TS, et al. The modified Bristow procedure for anterior shoulder instability: 26-year outcomes in Naval Academy midshipmen. Am J Sports Med 2006;34(5):778–86.
70. Warner JJ, Gill TJ, O'hollerhan JD, et al. Anatomical glenoid reconstruction for recurrent anterior glenohumeral instability with glenoid deficiency using an autogenous tricortical iliac crest bone graft. Am J Sports Med 2006;34(2): 205–12.
71. Weng PW, Shen HC, Lee HH, et al. Open reconstruction of large bony glenoid erosion with allogeneic bone graft for recurrent anterior shoulder dislocation. Am J Sports Med 2009;37(9):1792–7.
72. Provencher MT, Ghodadra N, LeClere L, et al. Anatomic osteochondral glenoid reconstruction for recurrent glenohumeral instability with glenoid deficiency using a distal tibia allograft. Arthroscopy 2009;25(4):446–52.

Surgical Management of Acromioclavicular Dislocations

Jay B. Cook, MD[a], John M. Tokish, MD[b],*

KEYWORDS

- Acromioclavicular dislocation • Anatomic reconstruction • Military population

KEY POINTS

- Acromioclavicular (AC) injuries are a common and disabling injury in a military population.
- Physical requirements often require a more aggressive treatment approach in this population.
- There is emerging research to support more anatomic reconstructions.
- In spite of these anatomic approaches, AC joint separations remain a challenging condition to treat.

INTRODUCTION

Epidemiology

Acromioclavicular (AC) separations are common injuries that recently have been the topic of increasing discussion in the literature. The incidence of AC injuries has been reported at 1.8 per 10,000 inhabitants per year in the general population.[1,2] Football players are at an increased risk of sustaining an injury to the AC joint and this risk increases with level of competition.[3,4] Similarly, an increased incidence has been reported in military populations up to 92 per 10,000 person years.[5] The AC ligamentous complex is critical to normal function of the shoulder girdle; disruption of these ligaments can lead to significant changes in shoulder mechanics and scapular dyskinesis, including a significant impact on activities such as bench press.[6–10]

Pertinent Anatomy

The AC joint is a diarthrodial joint with an intricate ligamentous complex that includes a dense capsule that surrounds the joint, in which is an intraarticular disk. Surrounding the capsule are the AC ligaments that provide the primary anterior-posterior (AP)

[a] Winn Army Community Hospital, 1061 Harmon Avenue, Fort Stewart, GA 31314, USA;
[b] Steadman Hawkins Clinic of the Carolinas, 200 Patewood C, Suite 100, Greenville SC 29615, USA
* Corresponding author. 25 Dove Drake Drive, Richmond Hill, GA 31324.
E-mail address: jtoke95@aol.com

Clin Sports Med 33 (2014) 721–737
http://dx.doi.org/10.1016/j.csm.2014.06.009
0278-5919/14/$ – see front matter © 2014 Elsevier Inc. All rights reserved.
sportsmed.theclinics.com

stabilization, in particular the posterior and superior portions.[11] Just medial to the AC joint are the coracoclavicular (CC) ligaments, which are the primary stabilizers to superior-inferior motion (**Fig. 1**).[11]

The anatomy of the AC joint complex has been thoroughly described. Earlier publications focused on specific length and measurements for the insertion points of the CC ligaments.[12–14] Rios and colleagues[15] performed an anatomic study that found similar absolute measurements of the ligament insertion point from the lateral end of the clavicle; however, they divided these by the clavicular length to establish a ratio, which was very consistent across all their specimens. The average ratios for the conoid and trapezoid tunnels were 0.24 and 0.17 respectively. Using this idea, Cook and colleagues[16] retrospectively reviewed 28 patients who had undergone anatomic CC ligament reconstructions and found that placement of the conoid tunnel medial to a ratio of 0.25 was a risk factor for early loss of reduction (**Fig. 2**).

Classification

The Rockwood classification is the most commonly used classification and is summarized in **Table 1**.[17] A single radiograph of both clavicles with a Zanca view should be used. The CC distance is then measured and compared with the contralateral side. In cases where the status of the CC ligaments is unclear, a weighted view may be obtained and the CC distance will significantly increase compared with the contralateral side if they have been disrupted. Posterior displacement and thus the diagnosis of a type IV, is best assessed on an axillary radiograph.

The "Optimal Technique"

A recent systematic review reported that more than 150 variations have been described to treat symptomatic AC joint separations.[18] One could conclude from this that there is currently no single technique that has been proven clearly superior to all others.[19] Techniques have included various pins, plates, screws, and suture constructs, many of which are still in use. The Weaver-Dunn procedure and modifications of it have been used since it was first described. Many new techniques and biomechanical studies still use the Weaver-Dunn as a comparison group.[20–23]

To date, no reconstruction technique can duplicate the stability and physiology of a native, intact AC joint complex. However, several biomechanical studies have

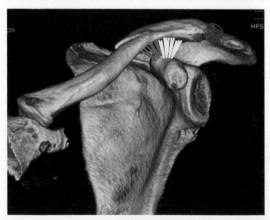

Fig. 1. The ligamentous complex surrounding the acromioclavicular joint. The acromioclavicular (*red*), trapezoid (*yellow*), and conoid (*blue*) ligaments are noted.

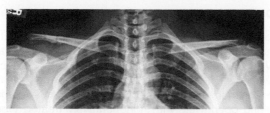

Fig. 2. Patient experienced an early loss of reduction before the first postoperative visit despite no reported trauma. Note the medialized clavicular bone tunnels.

supported further development and use of an anatomic reconstruction by demonstrating that the anatomic reconstruction comes closer to recreating natural stability than other surgical techniques.[24–28] Anatomic approaches, such as those described by Mazzocca and colleagues,[29] have shown promising early clinical results.[30]

Additionally, newer technology has allowed techniques to develop that use arthroscopic assistance. Suture buttons, such as the Tightrope (Arthrex Inc, Naples, FL, USA), have been used with an arthroscopic technique to treat acute injuries.[31,32] Salzmann and colleagues[33] drilled two tunnels in the clavicle and coracoid to recreate the CC ligaments in acute injuries. These hold the joint reduced until the native ligaments can heal. Biomechanical and medium-term follow-up has been reported with good success by these investigators.[32,34,35] Others have reported success with similar techniques.[20,31,36–39] The next progression was to incorporate a suture button to stabilize a chronic injury while allowing a biologic graft to incorporate. The Graftrope (Arthrex Inc, Naples, FL, USA) was a promising device designed for precisely this function; early results were good and there was strong biomechanical data to support its use.[20,26,40,41] However, subsequent studies demonstrated that the device often led to suboptimal outcomes.[42–44]

Although no optimal technique yet exists for the treatment of these injuries, there is continued clinical and biomechanical evidence in support of more anatomic reconstructions. The authors' current approach is a variation on anatomic reconstructions described by Mazzocca and colleagues[29] with several modifications.[30] First, we have found that an arthroscopic approach to the coracoid anatomy aids is a safe and accurate passage of the graft and allows the surgeon to address associated disease, which has been cited with up to a 30% incidence.[45–47] Second, the authors do not cross the limbs of the graft because doing so risks developing differential tension in one of the graft limbs. We prefer to ensure that the graft slides throughout its course to ensure equal tension in the limbs. Finally, we routinely run the trapezoid limb of the graft laterally to assist in the reconstruction of the AC joint capsule. We believe this helps support anteroposterior stability to the joint similar to the native anatomy.[11]

Table 1 Classification			
Type	**AC Ligament Status**	**CC Ligament Status**	**Displacement**
I	Partially torn	Intact	None
II	Disrupted	Intact	Minimal
III	Disrupted	Disrupted	<100% increase in CC distance
IV	Disrupted	Disrupted	Posterior through trapezius
V	Disrupted	Disrupted	>100% increase in CC distance
VI	Disrupted	Disrupted	Subacromial or subcoracoid

INDICATIONS AND CONTRAINDICATIONS

Indications and contraindications are summarized in **Table 2**. Traditionally, this algorithm as helped guide treatment because types I and II are usually treated conservatively and types IV, V, and VI are frequently treated operatively. Type III injuries have long been controversial.[19] There is evidence for approximately 80% good outcomes with nonoperative management of this injury.[6,48,49] A recent systematic review noted 14 studies comparing operatively with nonoperatively treated type III injuries with overall similar outcomes and a return to military duty in half the time for the nonoperatively group.[18] However, these data should be individualized because studies have noted that some activities, such as bench press, may not return to baseline.[6] In a military population in which pushups are an occupational necessity, such persistent deficits can have a tangible effect on the career and military readiness of soldiers. The authors have found that a significant portion of our type III AC joint separations fail conservative management. This finding is consistent with a study by Mulier and colleagues,[49] which reports that 17% of patients failed conservative management and required subsequent surgical treatment to achieve an optimal result.

The critical decision step is to determine which of the type III AC injuries are likely to fail nonoperative management. There is some evidence that chronic injuries do worse than those fixed acutely.[16,50–52] Therefore, those that present early after injury are carefully scrutinized (**Fig. 3**). In active patients who are less tolerant of an unstable joint, we perform stress radiographs to determine if there is further displacement under load. A cross-arm adducted radiograph, as described by Basmania, can reveal overlap of the acromion and clavicle in some AC separations, which has been suggested as further evidence of instability.[53] This is a modification of a techniques described by Alexander, in which the patient is asked to cross both arms, thrusting the shoulders forward, and a scapular Y view is taken of both shoulder for comparison of AC overlap.[54,55] More recently, horizontal stress radiographs have been shown to demonstrate instability that is independent of vertical displacement. The authors have used this technique to also evaluate higher risk patients for consideration of early operative intervention.[56,57] Although studies are lacking to validate these enhanced techniques, we have found the techniques helpful as a guide to determine which patients may ultimately benefit from earlier operative intervention.

SURGICAL TECHNIQUE OR PROCEDURE
Preoperative Planning

The AP radiograph or Zanca view should be used to preoperatively template the clavicle to ascertain the appropriate distances from the lateral edge of the clavicle

Table 2
Indications and contraindications for surgery

Indication	Contraindication
• High-grade injury (Types IV, V, VI)	• Low-grade injury (Type I, II)
• Failed nonoperative treatment (pain, weakness, fatigue, instability)	• Patient unable to comply with postoperative restrictions
• High risk of failing conservative management	• Patient needs early return to work or duty
• Polytrauma[62]	• Medical comorbidities precluding surgery
• Associated injury requiring operative treatment[63,64]	
• Open injury or skin at risk	
• Significant patient concern for cosmesis	

Algorithm for Acute Type III Injuries

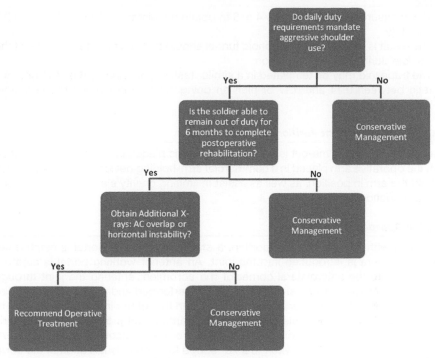

Fig. 3. Algorithm authors use to help determine which acute type III injuries are more likely to fail nonoperative treatment and should be surgically treated early. Additional radiographs can include bilateral stress Zanca views if not previously obtained, the Alexander view, cross-body adducted view, or axillary stress views.

for optimal tunnel placement. Templating at or just lateral to the anatomic centers of the trapezoid and conoid ligaments, at 17% and 24% of the clavicular length, respectively, has shown to be effective in preventing postoperative loss of reduction (**Fig. 4**).[6,16]

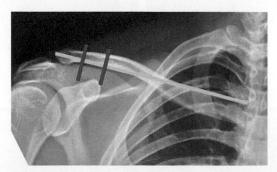

Fig. 4. Preoperative templating of the clavicular bone tunnels. The length of the clavicle is measured (*yellow line*) and the length is multiplied by the anatomic ratios of the conoid and trapezoid, 0.24 and 0.17, respectively. The optimal tunnel placement is at or just lateral to the anatomic ratios (*red lines*). These distances are then measured from the distal end of the clavicle to place the bone tunnel.

1. A measurement is made from the lateral to medial border of the clavicle in a straight line.
2. This measurement is divided by 4 or 5 to obtain the distance of a ratio between 0.2 and 0.25.
3. The result is the distance the conoid tunnel should be from the lateral border of the clavicle during the reconstruction.
4. The trapezoid may be templated in a similar fashion, dividing by 6 or 7 to obtain a ratio between 0.14 and 0.17 or plan on being 1.5 to 2 cm lateral to the conoid tunnel.

Preparation and Patient Positioning

After proper surgical time-out is taken, the patient is placed in a beach chair position with the operative arm placed in a commercial arm-holding device. This device serves to hold the arm in position, as well as assist in limiting gravity's effect on the AC joint during reduction and fixation.

Surgical Approach

Beginning with the arthroscopic portion, a standard posterior portal is established and the camera is introduced into the joint. An anterior working portal is created, just inferior to the anterolateral corner of the acromion, entering the joint through the rotator interval. A diagnostic arthroscopy is performed and any concomitant disease is addressed. An ablator is then used to open the rotator interval, taking care to avoid the superior and middle glenohumeral ligaments (**Fig. 5**). The subscapularis tendon may be followed medially until the base of the coracoid is encountered. At this point, the surgeon may switch to a 70° scope for better visualization of the coracoid undersurface, which is exposed using the ablator to remove all soft tissues from the medial to the lateral border (**Fig. 6**). The medial border of the coracoid should be clearly visualized. Neurovascular structures are usually 3 to 4 cm away. Surrounding fatty tissue may be encountered, which indicates adequate dissection has been obtained.[58]

A 3 to 4 cm, longitudinal incision is then made over the distal clavicle. The clavipectoral fascia is incised and dissection is carried down in a single flap through the

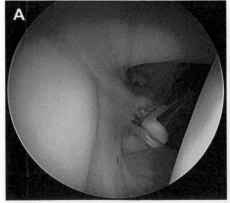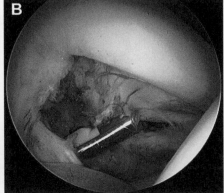

Fig. 5. (*A*) An ablator is used to open the rotator interval ensuring to avoid the superior and middle glenohumeral ligaments. (*B*) Dissection is carried medially following the subscapularis tendon.

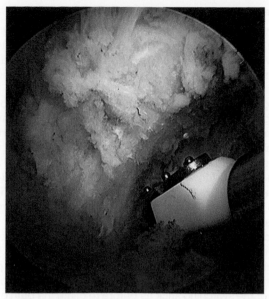

Fig. 6. The base of the coracoid is exposed to allow visualization of the medial and lateral border.

periosteum, which is elevated both anteriorly and posteriorly (**Fig. 7**). This partially releases and raises the trapezius and deltoid fascia in repairable flaps. The anterior and posterior borders of the clavicle are identified. The extent of the incision is dictated by visualization of the clavicle medially to allow placement of the conoid tunnel as determined with preoperative templating. Laterally, the incision is extended so that the trapezoid tunnel can be adequately drilled. Care must be taken to ensure the AC joint can be reduced. This often requires the removal of interposed soft tissue. In such cases, the incision should be extended laterally to expose the AC joint and tissue removed until the joint can be reduced adequately without undue pressure on the joint. The distal clavicle is not routinely excised except in cases in which reduction cannot be otherwise achieved.

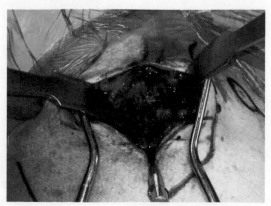

Fig. 7. Dissection is carried down to the clavicle with thick fascial flaps to facilitate closure. The AC joint was exposed in this approach.

Surgical Procedure

A ruler is used to measure from the lateral border of the clavicle and a marker or electrocautery is used to mark the position of the two bone tunnels on the clavicle based on the preoperative template. The conoid tunnel can be positioned slightly posterior and the trapezoid slightly anterior to midline. A 5 mm drill is then used to drill both tunnels bicortically.

A blunt switching stick is then used to create a path to the medial border of the coracoid. Until the surgeon is familiar with this, an anterior cruciate ligament–aiming guide may be used by introducing it through the anterior portal and placing it at the medial side of the coracoid under direct visualization with the arthroscope. The bullet on the guide may be placed either through the conoid tunnel, if the angle allows, or just anterior to the clavicle in line with the tunnel. The switching stick is then placed through the guide and manually advanced until visualized just medial to the coracoid (**Fig. 8**). The guide is then removed and a curette inserted through the anterior portal to protect the tip while a metal, cannulated, portal introducer is placed over the switching stick to dilate the path (**Fig. 9**). The curette and switching stick are removed and a stiff passing suture or suture-passing wire is placed through the introducer and retrieved out the anterior portal.

In a similar fashion, the blunt switching stick is used to create a path lateral to the coracoid either through the trapezoid tunnel or just anterior to the clavicle. The introducer is placed over the switching stick as before to dilate the path of the graft and the distal tip is protected using a curette. Once dilated, a ring grasper is used to retrieve the passing suture laterally. If the sutures are anterior to the clavicle, a suture lasso, suture passer, or similar device can be used through the bone tunnels to retrieve the suture from anterior. The suture is then toggled to ensure that is moves freely under the coracoid.

An autograft or nonirradiated allograft semitendinosus tendon is prepared with locking stitches on each end, and the passing suture is used to pull the lead sutures on the graft from medial to lateral through the bone tunnels. The graft is then pulled into place in a similar manner, looping under the coracoid (**Fig. 10**). The graft is then toggled, making certain that it can glide without restraint to allow even tension on the limbs.

The medial limb should be left long enough to reach just past the lateral tunnel. Then, a 4.5 or 5 mm interference screw is placed into the tunnel. The AC joint is then reduced fully by pressing down on the lateral edge of the clavicle with the metal

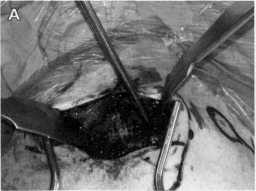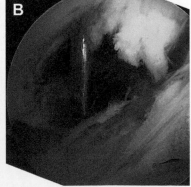

Fig. 8. (*A*) A switching stick is used to create a track from the clavicle to the medial border of the coracoid. In this patient, it is being inserted just anterior to the clavicle. (*B*) It is then seen protruding through the soft tissues medial to the coracoid.

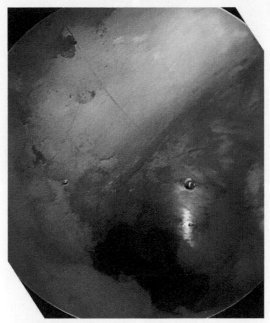

Fig. 9. The metal cannula introducer is used over the switching stick to dilate the track and is visualized medial to the coracoid.

cannula introducer and pushing up from under the elbow. While the reduction is held, the slack is pulled out via the lateral limb of the graft and a second interference screw is placed. The lateral limb should be long enough to cross the AC joint.

The excess medial limb is sutured to the lateral limb with a high strength, number 5 suture. The lateral limb is then brought superiorly across the AC joint on the posterior portion and secured to reinforce the posterosuperior AC ligament. This can be done by suturing to native tissue if it is present or by using a suture anchor.

Final arthroscopic inspection can be performed to ensure the graft is seated firmly on the undersurface of the coracoid (**Fig. 11**). The wounds are irrigated thoroughly. The flaps containing trapezial and deltoid fascia are sutured together over the repair using a number 1 suture, incorporating the graft on the superior surface of the AC joint. The remainder of the wound is closed in layered fashion and sterilely dressed. A radiograph may be taken in the operating room to confirm anatomic reduction of the AC joint.

POSTOPERATIVE CARE

Postoperatively, the shoulder is placed in a shoulder immobilizer and radiographs are taken in recovery that include an AP and modified axillary view. Between surgery and the first follow-up, the patient is only allowed to do pendulum exercises and is otherwise restricted to the shoulder immobilizer. Until 6 weeks postoperatively, the patient is only allowed passive motion in forward elevation and abduction, as well as internal and external rotation. Use of the sling is still encouraged to protect the repair. Between 6 and 12 weeks after surgery, the patient transitions to active motion and works with physical therapy to restore full motion while remaining non–weight bearing. Light isometric strengthening is begun in internal and external rotation. After 12 weeks, the

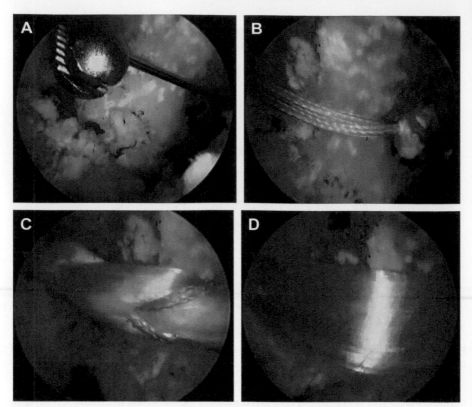

Fig. 10. (*A*) A grasper is used from the lateral track to retrieve the suture passing wire out the trapezoid tunnel. (*B*) The wire pulls the lead sutures on the graft out laterally. (*C*) These sutures are used to position the graft. (*D*) The arthroscope allows good visualization of the graft position under the coracoid.

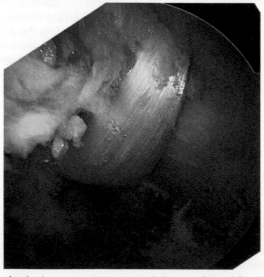

Fig. 11. The graft is checked once more to ensure it is securely and firmly seated around the coracoid.

patient is allowed to pursue strengthening with the goal to return to full objective strength by 16 weeks postoperatively. Emphasis is placed on scapular rhythm and balanced strengthening, as well as rotator cuff optimization.

At 4 to 5 months postoperatively, the patient is transitioned to functional and duty-specific activities, under the supervision of the therapist. Full return to unrestricted duty is typically allowed at 6 months.

COMPLICATIONS AND MANAGEMENT

The history of AC joint stabilization contains a colorful list of complications specific to the individual techniques used. This discussion focuses on those that are specific to recent anatomic reconstructions and are summarized in **Table 3**. Other, more infrequent complications can include adhesive capsulitis, neuropathy, distal clavicle hypertrophy, and AC joint pain, to name a few.

Complications are managed on a case-by-case basis. The most common in the authors' experiences is an early partial loss of reduction (**Fig. 12**). Despite radiographic appearance, these patients often have gone on to return to full duty and be asymptomatic without further intervention. Thus, a postoperative patient who returns with early partial loss of reduction is first managed conservatively with completion of postoperative rehabilitation. If still symptomatic, the patient is offered a revision reconstruction with either a similar technique (see above discussion) or with a tendon loop sutured to itself, similar to previous reports.[59,60] The authors have recently added a hook plate–type device in the treatment of all revisions and have found it helpful in supporting the reduction. The hook plate is removed between 3 and 4 months postoperatively to minimize the chance of further complications.[61]

Clavicle fractures can be treated with plating of the clavicle and, if necessary, revisions can be done in conjunction with the plates (**Fig. 13**). Coracoid fractures can occur, particularly in techniques involving a coracoid tunnel (**Fig. 14**). Often, these can be fixed with a single screw. Infections should be treated with antibiotics, irrigation, debridement, and revision as indicated by depth and severity of the infection. Other complications should be managed as indicated.

OUTCOMES

Most anatomic-type reconstructions have been reported as successful (**Table 4**). In a military population, return to unrestricted duty has been reported in up to 84% of patients using anatomic reconstructions.[16] However, there are several limitations to these studies. Most are not specific to an athletic population, have short-term follow-up, and do not include functional outcomes testing. Thus, their applicability to more active individual patients over longer periods of time needs further study.

Table 3 Complications	
Complication	**Incidence (Source)**
Loss of reduction (early or late)	Up to 29%[16]
Clavicle fracture	Up to 18%[43]
Infection	Up to 6%[30,43]
Hardware pain	Up to 4%[65]
Total complication rates	Up to 25%–30%[16,43,65]

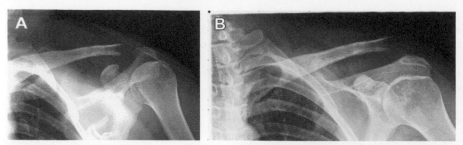

Fig. 12. (A) Immediate postoperative radiograph after an anatomic reconstruction. (B) Loss of reduction noted at the first postoperative visit. The patient completed the postoperative therapy and went on to be asymptomatic and return to full duty as an infantryman.

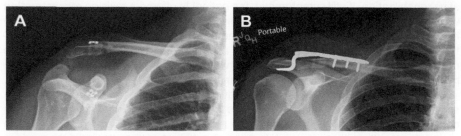

Fig. 13. (A) Radiographs taken at the first postoperative visit demonstrated loss of reduction and a distal clavicle fracture through one of the bone tunnels. (B) The patient was revised with an allograft and a hook plate for supplemental stabilization.

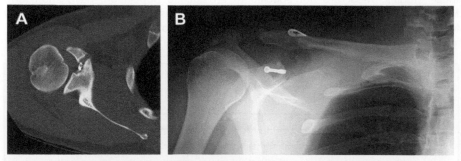

Fig. 14. (A) The patient sustained a coracoid fracture through the tunnel drilled for the suture button through the coracoid. (B) The fracture was fixed with a longitudinal screw.

Table 4
Outcomes of anatomic reconstructions

Study	Patients	Follow-up (Average)	Subjective Satisfaction (Average)	Objective Scores
Tauber et al,[21] 2009	12	37 mo	9.6 out of 10	ASES 96 Constant 93
Fraschini et al,[66] 2010	30	15 mo	93%	UCLA 28.4
Carofino & Mazzocca,[30] 2010	17	21 mo	SANE 94.4	ASES 92 SST 11.8 Constant 94.7
Ladermann et al,[67] 2011	37	4.5 y	95%	Constant 96 DASH 7
Martetschlager et al,[65] 2013	43[a]	2.4 y	9 out of 10 SANE 89	ASES 91 QuickDASH 7

Abbreviations: ASES, American Shoulder Elbow Surgery; DASH, Disabilities of the Arm, Shoulder and Hand; SST, Simple Shoulder Test; UCLA, University of California Los Angeles.
[a] Only reported on subjects without a complication.

SUMMARY

AC injuries are common in the military population. Many AC injuries can be treated conservatively with good success. Due to requirements of a military population, however, conservative management may fail at a higher rate than in civilian populations. Surgical management is indicated for high-grade injuries and those that are refractory to nonoperative treatment, as well as in those patients at high risk for failure of conservative management. Many techniques exist and there is no single superior technique. The anatomic reconstruction is evolving into a more consistent procedure with good biomechanical support. However, complication rates and failures are higher than ideal; thus, the surgeon must approach this injury with meticulous attention to detail and technique.

Pearls and pitfalls of arthroscopic reconstruction technique

Pearls	Pitfalls
• Using a shaver or a liberator may facilitate exposure of the coracoid if soft tissue occludes visualization.	• Placement of bone tunnels too far anteriorly or posteriorly, or in too close of proximity, risks clavicle fractures.[18,30]
• Careful dissection of the distal clavicle with thick flaps will allow additional soft tissue coverage during closure.	• If using a coracoid tunnel, care should be taken to ensure that it is center-center to decrease risk of fracture.[69]
• When placing the switching stick, aim for the coracoid and "walk" it medially or laterally until it is visualized at the border of the coracoid.	• Do not rely on assessment of the adequacy of the reduction by palpation of the AC joint through the skin. Do not hesitate to extend the incision laterally to directly visualize reduction or use intraoperative fluoroscopy.
• A suture button can be used for augmentation of the fixation through the coracoid; this should be passed before the graft.[68]	
• Choose an interference screw long enough be bicortical to maximize fixation.	

REFERENCES

1. Chillemi C, Franceschini V, Dei Giudici L, et al. Epidemiology of isolated acromioclavicular joint dislocation. Emerg Med Int 2013;2013:171609.
2. Simovitch R, Sanders B, Ozbaydar M, et al. Acromioclavicular joint injuries: diagnosis and management. J Am Acad Orthop Surg 2009;17(4):207–19.
3. Lynch TS, Saltzman MD, Ghodasra JH, et al. Acromioclavicular joint injuries in the national football league: epidemiology and management. Am J Sports Med 2013;41(12):2904–8.
4. Dragoo JL, Braun HJ, Bartlinski SE, et al. Acromioclavicular joint injuries in National Collegiate Athletic Association football: data from the 2004-2005 through 2008-2009 National Collegiate Athletic Association Injury Surveillance System. Am J Sports Med 2012;40(9):2066–71.
5. Pallis M, Cameron KL, Svoboda SJ, et al. Epidemiology of acromioclavicular joint injury in young athletes. Am J Sports Med 2012;40(9):2072–7.
6. Schlegel TF, Burks RT, Marcus RL, et al. A prospective evaluation of untreated acute grade III acromioclavicular separations. Am J Sports Med 2001;29(6):699–703.
7. Gumina S, Carbone S, Postacchini F. Scapular dyskinesis and SICK scapula syndrome in patients with chronic type III acromioclavicular dislocation. Arthroscopy 2009;25(1):40–5.
8. Oki S, Matsumura N, Iwamoto W, et al. The function of the acromioclavicular and coracoclavicular ligaments in shoulder motion: a whole-cadaver study. Am J Sports Med 2012;40(11):2617–26.
9. Oki S, Matsumura N, Iwamoto W, et al. Acromioclavicular joint ligamentous system contributing to clavicular strut function: a cadaveric study. J Shoulder Elbow Surg 2013;22(10):1433–9.
10. Murena L, Canton G, Vulcano E, et al. Scapular dyskinesis and SICK scapula syndrome following surgical treatment of type III acute acromioclavicular dislocations. Knee Surg Sports Traumatol Arthrosc 2013;21(5):1146–50.
11. Fukuda K, Craig EV, An KN, et al. Biomechanical study of the ligamentous system of the acromioclavicular joint. J Bone Joint Surg Am 1986;68(3):434–40.
12. Boehm TD, Kirschner S, Fischer A, et al. The relation of the coracoclavicular ligament insertion to the acromioclavicular joint: a cadaver study of relevance to lateral clavicle resection. Acta Orthop Scand 2003;74(6):718–21.
13. Harris RI, Vu DH, Sonnabend DH, et al. Anatomic variance of the coracoclavicular ligaments. J Shoulder Elbow Surg 2001;10(6):585–8.
14. Renfree KJ, Riley MK, Wheeler D, et al. Ligamentous anatomy of the distal clavicle. J Shoulder Elbow Surg 2003;12(4):355–9.
15. Rios CG, Arciero RA, Mazzocca AD. Anatomy of the clavicle and coracoid process for reconstruction of the coracoclavicular ligaments. Am J Sports Med 2007;35(5):811–7.
16. Cook JB, Shaha JS, Rowles DJ, et al. Clavicular bone tunnel malposition leads to early failures in coracoclavicular ligament reconstructions. Am J Sports Med 2013;41(1):142–8.
17. Rockwood CA Jr. Injuries to the acromioclavicular joint. In: Rockwood CA Jr, editor. Fractures in adults. 2nd edition. Philadelphia: JB Lippincott; 1984. p. 860–910.
18. Beitzel K, Cote MP, Apostolakos J, et al. Current concepts in the treatment of acromioclavicular joint dislocations. Arthroscopy 2013;29(2):387–97.
19. Johansen JA, Grutter PW, McFarland EG, et al. Acromioclavicular joint injuries: indications for treatment and treatment options. J Shoulder Elbow Surg 2011; 20(2 Suppl):S70–82.

20. Beitzel K, Obopilwe E, Chowaniec DM, et al. Biomechanical comparison of arthroscopic repairs for acromioclavicular joint instability: suture button systems without biological augmentation. Am J Sports Med 2011;39(10):2218–25.
21. Tauber M, Gordon K, Koller H, et al. Semitendinosus tendon graft versus a modified Weaver-Dunn procedure for acromioclavicular joint reconstruction in chronic cases: a prospective comparative study. Am J Sports Med 2009;37(1):181–90.
22. Lee SJ, Keefer EP, McHugh MP, et al. Cyclical loading of coracoclavicular ligament reconstructions: a comparative biomechanical study. Am J Sports Med 2008;36(10):1990–7.
23. Lee SJ, Nicholas SJ, Akizuki KH, et al. Reconstruction of the coracoclavicular ligaments with tendon grafts: a comparative biomechanical study. Am J Sports Med 2003;31(5):648–55.
24. Costic RS, Labriola JE, Rodosky MW, et al. Biomechanical rationale for development of anatomical reconstructions of coracoclavicular ligaments after complete acromioclavicular joint dislocations. Am J Sports Med 2004;32(8):1929–36.
25. Mazzocca AD, Spang JT, Rodriguez RR, et al. Biomechanical and radiographic analysis of partial coracoclavicular ligament injuries. Am J Sports Med 2008; 36(7):1397–402.
26. Thomas K, Litsky A, Jones G, et al. Biomechanical comparison of coracoclavicular reconstructive techniques. Am J Sports Med 2011;39(4):804–10.
27. Yoo YS, Tsai AG, Ranawat AS, et al. A biomechanical analysis of the native coracoclavicular ligaments and their influence on a new reconstruction using a coracoid tunnel and free tendon graft. Arthroscopy 2010;26(9):1153–61.
28. Grutter PW, Petersen SA. Anatomical acromioclavicular ligament reconstruction: a biomechanical comparison of reconstructive techniques of the acromioclavicular joint. Am J Sports Med 2005;33(11):1723–8.
29. Mazzocca AD, Conway JE, Johnson S, et al. The anatomic coracoclavicular ligament reconstruction. Oper Tech Sports Med 2004;12(1):6.
30. Carofino BC, Mazzocca AD. The anatomic coracoclavicular ligament reconstruction: surgical technique and indications. J Shoulder Elbow Surg 2010; 19(2 Suppl):37–46.
31. Scheibel M, Droschel S, Gerhardt C, et al. Arthroscopically assisted stabilization of acute high-grade acromioclavicular joint separations. Am J Sports Med 2011; 39(7):1507–16.
32. Venjakob AJ, Salzmann GM, Gabel F, et al. Arthroscopically assisted 2-bundle anatomic reduction of acute acromioclavicular joint separations: 58-month findings. Am J Sports Med 2013;41(3):615–21.
33. Salzmann GM, Walz L, Schoettle PB, et al. Arthroscopic anatomical reconstruction of the acromioclavicular joint. Acta Orthop Belg 2008;74(3):397–400.
34. Salzmann GM, Walz L, Buchmann S, et al. Arthroscopically assisted 2-bundle anatomical reduction of acute acromioclavicular joint separations. Am J Sports Med 2010;38(6):1179–87.
35. Walz L, Salzmann GM, Fabbro T, et al. The anatomic reconstruction of acromioclavicular joint dislocations using 2 TightRope devices: a biomechanical study. Am J Sports Med 2008;36(12):2398–406.
36. Glanzmann MC, Buchmann S, Audige L, et al. Clinical and radiographical results after double flip button stabilization of acute grade III and IV acromioclavicular joint separations. Arch Orthop Trauma Surg 2013;133(12):1699–707.
37. Beris A, Lykissas M, Kostas-Agnantis I, et al. Management of acute acromioclavicular joint dislocation with a double-button fixation system. Injury 2013. [Epub ahead of print].

38. Defoort S, Verborgt O. Functional and radiological outcome after arthroscopic and open acromioclavicular stabilization using a double-button fixation system. Acta Orthop Belg 2010;76(5):585–91.

39. Murena L, Vulcano E, Ratti C, et al. Arthroscopic treatment of acute acromioclavicular joint dislocation with double flip button. Knee Surg Sports Traumatol Arthrosc 2009;17(12):1511–5.

40. DeBerardino TM, Pensak MJ, Ferreira J, et al. Arthroscopic stabilization of acromioclavicular joint dislocation using the AC graftrope system. J Shoulder Elbow Surg 2010;19(2 Suppl):47–52.

41. Geaney LE, Miller MD, Ticker JB, et al. Management of the failed AC joint reconstruction: causation and treatment. Sports Med Arthrosc 2010;18(3): 167–72.

42. Cook JB, Shaha JS, Rowles DJ, et al. Early failures with single clavicular transosseous coracoclavicular ligament reconstruction. J Shoulder Elbow Surg 2012; 21(12):1746–52.

43. Milewski MD, Tompkins M, Giugale JM, et al. Complications related to anatomic reconstruction of the coracoclavicular ligaments. Am J Sports Med 2012;40(7): 1628–34.

44. Gerhardt DC, VanDerWerf JD, Rylander LS, et al. Postoperative coracoid fracture after transcoracoid acromioclavicular joint reconstruction. J Shoulder Elbow Surg 2011;20(5):e6–10.

45. Tischer T, Salzmann GM, El-Azab H, et al. Incidence of associated injuries with acute acromioclavicular joint dislocations types III through V. Am J Sports Med 2009;37(1):136–9.

46. Pauly S, Gerhardt C, Haas NP, et al. Prevalence of concomitant intraarticular lesions in patients treated operatively for high-grade acromioclavicular joint separations. Knee Surg Sports Traumatol Arthrosc 2009;17(5):513–7.

47. Arrigoni P, Brady PC, Zottarelli L, et al. Associated lesions requiring additional surgical treatment in grade 3 acromioclavicular joint dislocations. Arthroscopy 2014;30(1):6–10.

48. Tibone J, Sellers R, Tonino P. Strength testing after third-degree acromioclavicular dislocations. Am J Sports Med 1992;20(3):328–31.

49. Mulier T, Stuyck J, Fabry G. Conservative treatment of acromioclavicular dislocation. Evaluation of functional and radiological results after six years follow-up. Acta Orthop Belg 1993;59(3):255–62.

50. Weinstein DM, McCann PD, McIlveen SJ, et al. Surgical treatment of complete acromioclavicular dislocations. Am J Sports Med 1995;23(3):324–31.

51. Rolf O, Hann von Weyhern A, Ewers A, et al. Acromioclavicular dislocation Rockwood III-V: results of early versus delayed surgical treatment. Arch Orthop Trauma Surg 2008;128(10):1153–7.

52. Dumontier C, Sautet A, Man M, et al. Acromioclavicular dislocations: treatment by coracoacromial ligamentoplasty. J Shoulder Elbow Surg 1995;4(2): 130–4.

53. Bontempo NA, Mazzocca AD. Biomechanics and treatment of acromioclavicular and sternoclavicular joint injuries. Br J Sports Med 2010;44(5):361–9.

54. Alexander OM. Dislocation of the acromioclavicular joint. Radiography 1949; 15(179):260 illust.

55. Alexander OM. Radiography of the acromioclavicular articulation. Med Radiogr Photogr 1954;30(2):34–9.

56. Wellmann M, da Silva G, Lichtenberg S, et al. Instabilitatsmuster bei Akromioklavikulargelenkverletzungen vom Typ Rockwood III: Bedeutung der horizontalen

Instabilitat. [Instability pattern of acromioclavicular joint dislocations type Rockwood III: relevance of horizontal instability]. Orthopade 2013;42(4):271–7 [in German].

57. Tauber M, Koller H, Hitzl W, et al. Dynamic radiologic evaluation of horizontal instability in acute acromioclavicular joint dislocations. Am J Sports Med 2010;38(6):1188–95.

58. Lo IK, Burkhart SS, Parten PM. Surgery about the coracoid: neurovascular structures at risk. Arthroscopy 2004;20(6):591–5.

59. Nicholas SJ, Lee SJ, Mullaney MJ, et al. Clinical outcomes of coracoclavicular ligament reconstructions using tendon grafts. Am J Sports Med 2007;35(11): 1912–7.

60. Yoo JC, Ahn JH, Yoon JR, et al. Clinical results of single-tunnel coracoclavicular ligament reconstruction using autogenous semitendinosus tendon. Am J Sports Med 2010;38(5):950–7.

61. Modi CS, Beazley J, Zywiel MG, et al. Controversies relating to the management of acromioclavicular joint dislocations. Bone Joint J 2013;95-B(12):1595–602.

62. Gallay SH, Hupel TM, Beaton DE, et al. Functional outcome of acromioclavicular joint injury in polytrauma patients. J Orthop Trauma 1998;12(3):159–63.

63. Woolf SK, Valentine BJ, Barfield WR, et al. Middle-third clavicle fracture with associated type IV acromioclavicular separation: case report and literature review. J Surg Orthop Adv 2013;22(2):183–6.

64. Beytemur O, Adanir O, Dincel YM, et al. Clavicle diaphyseal fracture, ipsilateral type 3 acromioclavicular joint dislocation stabilized with double plate. Int J Shoulder Surg 2013;7(4):153–4.

65. Martetschlager F, Horan MP, Warth RJ, et al. Complications after anatomic fixation and reconstruction of the coracoclavicular ligaments. Am J Sports Med 2013;41(12):2896–903.

66. Fraschini G, Ciampi P, Scotti C, et al. Surgical treatment of chronic acromioclavicular dislocation: comparison between two surgical procedures for anatomic reconstruction. Injury 2010;41(11):1103–6.

67. Ladermann A, Grosclaude M, Lubbeke A, et al. Acromioclavicular and coracoclavicular cerclage reconstruction for acute acromioclavicular joint dislocations. J Shoulder Elbow Surg 2011;20(3):401–8.

68. Cook JB, Tokish JM, Yim D, et al. Coracoclavicular ligament reconstruction: an arthroscopically assisted technique using biologic and synthetic fixation. Curr Orthop Pract 2013;24(5):5.

69. Ferreira JV, Chowaniec D, Obopilwe E, et al. Biomechanical evaluation of effect of coracoid tunnel placement on load to failure of fixation during repair of acromioclavicular joint dislocations. Arthroscopy 2012;28(9):1230–6.

Pectoralis Major Injuries
Evaluation and Treatment

Chad A. Haley, MD[a],*, Michael A. Zacchilli, MD[b]

KEYWORDS

- Pectoralis major muscle • Tendon rupture • Tendon tear • Tendon repair
- Cortical button

KEY POINTS

- The pectoralis major muscle has a clavicular head and a sternal head, with the sternal head inserting more proximal and posterior to the clavicular head.
- Pectoralis major tears typically occur from a rapid eccentric load, commonly during the flat bench press exercise.
- Surgical repair, ideally in an acute (<6 weeks) period, yields superior outcomes to nonoperative treatment in young, active individuals.
- Tendon to tendon, bone trough, suture anchor, and cortical button are effective techniques to repair pectoralis major tears.

INTRODUCTION

Pectoralis major (PM) tendon tears are relatively rare injuries that most commonly occur in the 20- to 40 year-old male athlete engaged in weight-lifting exercises, such as when performing a bench press. The tendon typically tears near its insertion during an eccentric contraction of the PM under heavy loads with the arm in extension and external rotation. An accurate and timely diagnosis of a PM tear is important because most studies report better outcomes with acute surgical repair. This article describes the anatomy of the PM muscle, injury epidemiology, tear classification, diagnosis including physical examination and imaging, treatment options for both nonoperative and operative management, complications, a review of the literature including military-related studies, and the authors' preferred technique.

ANATOMY
Muscle Architecture

The PM is a broad muscle generally described as having 2 distinct heads, the uniform clavicular and the segmented sternocostal.[1,2] The sternocostal head is described as

Disclosures: None.
[a] Department of Surgery, Keller Army Community Hospital, Building 900, West Point, NY 10996, USA; [b] Department of Orthopaedics and Rehabilitation, Womack Army Medical Center, 2817 Reilly Road, Fort Bragg, NC 28310, USA
* Corresponding author.
E-mail address: chad.a.haley.mil@mail.mil

Clin Sports Med 33 (2014) 739–756
http://dx.doi.org/10.1016/j.csm.2014.06.005
0278-5919/14/$ – see front matter Published by Elsevier Inc.

sportsmed.theclinics.com

having as few as 2 and as many as 7 segments.[1–3] Whereas some investigators describe the lowest portions of the muscle as a distinct abdominal segment of the sternocostal head,[3] others describe it as a separate head entirely.[4] Regardless of nomenclature, the most inferior muscle segments are usually described as reflecting posteriorly,[2] or cradling the adjacent superior muscle segment near their costal origin,[1] creating an inferior fold or "J" configuration when viewed in cross section.

Tendon Configuration

The extramuscular PM tendon can measure as little as 5 to 15 mm in medial-lateral length from the end of the myotendinous junction to the humeral insertion,[5] while overall tendon fiber length including the intramuscular portion averages 5 to 6 cm in medial-lateral length and 4 to 5 cm in proximal-distal width.[1,6] The humeral footprint is located on the lateral lip of the bicipital groove, begins approximately 4 cm distal to the tip of the greater tuberosity,[7] and measures approximately 4.8 to 7.7 cm in width (proximal-distal) and 1.4 to 5.6 mm in thickness (**Fig. 1**).[1,5–8] Klepps and colleagues[6] importantly documented significantly decreased tendon width after surgical disruption of the native insertion (5.7 cm attached, 4 cm detached), consistent with the clinical observations of the authors. The tendon is usually described as bilaminar in nature with continuity between the 2 laminae distally.[1,4] The relationship of the muscle proper to the tendinous insertion is described by some as a 90°[3] or 180°[5] twist, whereas others maintain that there is no twisting but rather overlapping insertion of individual laminae.[1] Clavicular head fibers course in parallel fashion and insert most distally at the humeral insertion, and comprise either all[3,5] or most of the anterior tendon lamina.[1] Most investigators describe a variable number of superior sternocostal segments as either contributing to the distal anterior tendon lamina[1] or forming a distinct middle lamina at the distal extent of the insertion.[3]

To summarize, in the authors' opinion reported differences are primarily a conflict of semantics attempting to describe one important relationship: the clavicular head and a variable portion of the superior sternocostal head comprise the anterior and inferior tendon fibers at the humeral insertion as 1 to 2 laminae, the manubrial portions of the sternocostal head comprise the nadir of the U-shaped insertion with variable connectivity to the anterior and posterior lamina, and the remaining segments of the sternocostal head insert posteriorly and superiorly, establishing the posterior limb of the "U."

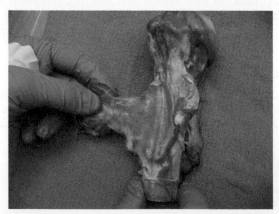

Fig. 1. The pectoralis major (PM) tendon inserts into the lateral edge of the bicipital groove, beginning 4 cm distal to the tip of the greater tuberosity with an insertional width of 4.8 to 7.7 cm and a thickness of 1.4 to 5.6 mm. (*Courtesy of* Brett D. Owens, MD, West Point, NY.)

Innervation

The PM muscle is supplied by C5-T1 nerve roots via the medial and lateral pectoral nerves, whose names are derived from the brachial plexus cord of origin.[2] The lateral pectoral nerve is generally described as supplying the clavicular head and upper segments of the sternocostal head.[2] After exiting the lateral cord of the brachial plexus from a variable location, the lateral pectoral nerve courses anterior to the axillary artery and medial to the pectoralis minor. It then accompanies the pectoral branches of the thoracoacromial arch in a distal course on the posterior surface of the proximal PM, entering the muscle at a mean 12.5 cm (95% confidence interval [CI] 10.0–14.9) medial to the humeral insertion.[2,6]

The medial pectoral nerve arises from the medial cord posterior to the axillary artery as 1 or 2 branches, which either pierce the pectoralis minor near the midclavicular line or travel lateral to the pectoralis minor (25%) as the nerves course distally. At least 1 branch will pierce the pectoralis minor in 62% to 75% of cases.[2,6] The nerve enters the undersurface of the PM in 2 to 3 branches[2] at a mean 11.9 cm (95% CI 8.6–15.3) medial to the humeral insertion and 2 cm proximal to the inferior edge,[6] innervating the lower sternocostal segments.

The safe zone for PM mobilization was described by Klepps and colleagues[6] in a cadaveric study for pectoralis transfer, and is located lateral to the pectoralis minor for a distance along the muscle of up to 8.5 cm from the humeral insertion. Vigilance is recommended in mobilization of the inferior PM border, owing to the proximity of the medial pectoral nerve insertion as already described.

Biomechanics

The main functions of the PM muscle are adduction, forward elevation (clavicular head), and internal rotation (sternocostal head). Whereas most human muscles have uniform muscle fiber lengths, the PM demonstrates significant variation across segments.[1,3,9] This configuration allows the PM to maximize power production through a broad range of muscle-shortening velocities but also results in disproportionately high fiber excursion in the inferior sternocostal head segments between 0° and 30° of extension.[3] This phenomenon is the proposed biomechanical cause of failure/rupture of the PM when maximal force is applied in a position of mechanical disadvantage (eg, bench press). Providers with experience in treating this injury are likely to recognize the commonality of this position of risk in a wide range of injury mechanisms.

INJURY EPIDEMIOLOGY

According to a 2012 meta-analysis, a total of 365 cases of PM rupture were reported in the medical literature between 1822 and 2010, with 76% reported after 1990.[9] There are no available prospective studies to define incidence in the general population. However, in an at-risk active duty US Army population, White and colleagues[10] demonstrated 7 pectoralis ruptures for 93,224 person-years of active-duty military service exposure. These injuries represented 14% of all major tendon ruptures in this population, with a rate of 1 per 13,317 person-years at risk.

Tears occur almost exclusively in active men in their third to fourth decades of life.[9,11–13] Approximately 75% of cases are related directly to sports activity. Weight-lifting exercises account for nearly 50% of cases reported in the literature,[9,11] with wrestling, jujitsu, and gymnastics also frequently implicated.[9,11,13,14]

Information describing the acuity of diagnosis and treatment in PM injuries is under-reported and/or variably defined, but 62% of published cases are labeled acute by investigators.[9] Tears occur primarily at the tendon insertion (59%–65%) and musculotendinous junction (24%–29%).[9,11] Classification of tear severity is often not provided, but 56% of published injuries are described as complete tears or avulsions.[9] It is the authors' opinion that publication bias may play a role in overestimating the proportion of complete tears. In their 2000 meta-analysis, Bak and colleagues[11] limited evaluation of tear severity to surgically confirmed published cases (91% complete), a statistic represented in an important 2010 review article.[13]

De Castro Pochini reported anabolic steroid use in more than 90% of patients in their 2014 case series of 60 complete ruptures,[15] and Aarima and colleagues[12] endorsed a rate of at least 36% in their 33-patient operative series, but its prevalence is otherwise infrequently reported in the literature overall.[11] Possible explanations for increased risk of tendon rupture in those exposed to anabolic steroids have been attributed to stiffening of the tendon and disproportionate gains in maximal force production.[11–13,15,16]

CLASSIFICATION

Tietjen[17] proposed an anatomic classification for PM injuries in 1980 with recommended treatment implications (**Table 1**). The classification was well suited to prevailing opinion at that time, with a more stringent indication for surgical intervention. It does not account for several variables now considered to have significant clinical implications, such as acuity, gradation of partial tears, and distinction between clavicular and sternocostal head injuries. These characteristics carry important implications in treatment and outcome.

The recent meta-analysis by ElMaraghy and Devereaux[9] has highlighted deficits in the quality of medical literature for PM ruptures. Imprecise description of injury anatomy and a paucity of information regarding acuity of diagnosis and treatment are common. These investigators proposed a comprehensive classification system (**Fig. 2**). It is a testament to the complexity of the anatomy that even within this comprehensive classification there is a noticeable deficit in quantitative description of the width of injuries, which are defined only by a qualitative "complete" or "incomplete."

DIAGNOSIS

Diagnosis should rely on a comprehensive history and physical examination in addition to imaging modalities. Treatment decisions, as outlined in herein, frequently depend on determination of complete versus partial tears. Even in the peer-reviewed literature, these terms are ill defined and their implications potentially contradictory when

Table 1
Tietjen classification of pectoralis major injuries

Type	Subtype	Description	Recommended Treatment
I	Sprain or contusion		Nonoperative
II	Partial tears		Nonoperative
III	Complete		Nonoperative
III	A	Sternoclavicular origin	Nonoperative
III	B	Muscle belly	Nonoperative
III	C	Musculotendinous junction	Operative for severe cosmetic/functional deformity
III	D	Insertion	Operative

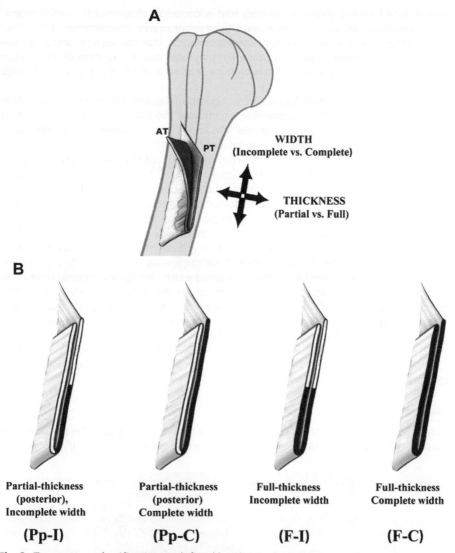

Fig. 2. Tear pattern classification as defined by ElMaraghy. (*A*) Demonstration of the bilaminar tendinous insertion, with the anterior tendon composed primarily of fibers from the clavicular head, and the posterior tendon composed of the sternocostal segments inserting more proximally at the lateral edge of the bicipital groove. (*B*) Partial tear patterns can be difficult to describe, with variable involvement of one or both lamina. (*From* ElMaraghy AW, Devereaux MW. A systematic review and comprehensive classification of pectoralis major tears. J Shoulder Elbow Surg 2012;21:412–22; with permission from Elsevier.)

considered relative to the PM anatomy.[9] The authors therefore consider it imperative that imaging modalities do not supersede the physical examination and clinical judgment, but rather augment medical decision making.

Physical Examination

Physical examination of acute PM ruptures often demonstrates significant swelling and hematomas of the anterior chest wall, axilla, and arm. Tenderness over the humeral insertion and along the axillary fold is common. Asymmetric medial prominence of the muscle belly may represent either hematoma or medialization of the muscle belly (**Fig. 3**). However, these signs are nonspecific, develop rapidly, and may take several weeks to resolve. More importantly, they limit direct palpation of the tendon and visualization of the axillary fold, which have been 2 of the most reliable findings in the authors' experience.

Examination of the axillary fold and direct comparison with the contralateral limb is performed while the patient isometrically contracts the PM in attempted adduction while resting the palms on the iliac crests. The fold is then visualized. Frequently there will be thinning, hollowing, or complete loss of the fold.[3,13]

In chronic cases cicatricial fibrosis, a prominent skin fold, webbing, and prominence of the distal deltoid insertion have all been described.[3,14] The examiner must take care to palpate the thickness of the suspected tendon by pinching the axillary fold, as the fascial sheath can mimic a visibly normal fold and delay diagnosis.[16,18] In patients with an athletic habitus, palpation is often easily performed for 5 to 6 cm proximal to the inferior border of the fold, and can assist in determining tears of complete versus incomplete width. Full-thickness tears are distinguished from partial-thickness tears by the presence of a distinct gap or defect (full thickness) as opposed to partial thinning (partial thickness) relative to the uninvolved extremity. Some investigators have described the visual "triangle sign" in cases of sternocostal rupture with an intact clavicular head.[15] In addition, with forward elevation, lateral inspection may demonstrate a visible retracted stump within the anterior axillary fold, termed the "S" sign.[14] The muscle belly itself should be palpated directly in a lateral to medial direction to identify muscle belly or origin defects. Finally, subjective strength examination in adduction, forward flexion, and internal rotation is performed with assessment for concomitant discomfort.

Plain Radiographs

Plain radiographs are of limited use in PM muscle ruptures, but should be performed to rule out additional abnormality and assess for the rare bony avulsion injury that occurs

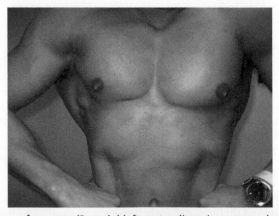

Fig. 3. Clinical image of an acute (2 weeks) left pectoralis major rupture demonstrate swelling and medialization of the muscle belly. Ecchymosis has resolved. Also noted is a "dropped nipple sign" as described by Funk. (*Courtesy of* Brett D. Owens, MD, West Point, NY; and *Data from* Funk L. Pectoralis major rupture—footprint technique. Produced by Wrightington Hospital. Available at: http://www.vumedi.com/video/pectoralis-major-rupture-footprint-technique/. Accessed March 1, 2014.)

2% to 5% of cases.[9,11] Attention to the glenohumeral joint should not be neglected if warranted by physical examination, as simultaneous shoulder dislocation and PM rupture has been described.[19] Examination of the muscle contour within the fold may be useful in some cases, and is more easily performed with modern digital radiographs.

Ultrasonography

The use of ultrasonography in identifying and describing PM tears has been documented and continues to evolve.[20–23] Pavlik and colleagues,[21] in 1998, were the first to report use of ultrasonography as the primary imaging modality used to successfully diagnosis pectoralis tears in 2 patients. Bak and colleagues[11] described a diagnosis of a chronic bony avulsion tear (10 months) in a delayed consult with no reported prior plain radiographs. Its use has previously been recommended by some investigators to allow more rapid diagnosis and treatment. Though less expensive and often more rapidly accessible than magnetic resonance imaging (MRI), ultrasonography is highly operator dependent. Two recent studies have evaluated sonographic correlation with surgical findings. Weaver and colleagues[22] published a descriptive sonographic case series of PM ruptures, which does little to define the role or accuracy of the examination. In 2013, Lee and colleagues[23] performed a retrospective correlative study motivated by the concerns of 6 experienced musculoskeletal fellowship trained radiologists. Of 22 PM tears diagnosed sonographically, 9 studies performed a mean 31 days after injury had surgical correlation available and were reviewed. The 9 reviewed cases demonstrated typical demographics. Surgical evaluations had revealed 6 cases of insertional sternocostal head rupture while 3 were complete insertional ruptures of both heads. In no case was there a complete absence of tendon or tendon-like tissue. In 3 cases (50% of the partial-thickness, complete-width tears), a normal distal tendon was visualized. In 6 cases (including all full-thickness, complete-width tears) linear thickened hypoechoic tissue was interpreted by the investigators as injured but intact tendon. Hypoechoic fluid was identified at the musculotendinous junction in 8 of 9 cases. The investigators therefore disclosed concern that the use of ultrasonography to diagnose PM tears is prone to false-negative results in complete tears, and may lead to incorrect localization of insertional avulsions as musculotendinous injuries.[23] The utility of ultrasonography as a reliable imaging modality is therefore brought into question by recent research.

Magnetic Resonance Imaging

MRI was reported as a successfully diagnostic imaging modality for PM ruptures in the early 1990s,[19,24,25] but also had at least one documented failure in the diagnosis of a complete chronic tear.[26] In the largest PM study of its time, Bak and colleagues[11] questioned the reliability of MRI, owing to the absence of correlative studies.

Three correlation studies were performed between March 1999 and May 2000.[5,27,28] All 3 studies used 1.5-T magnets and recommended small field-of-view, thin-cut (3 mm) series in axial and oblique coronal planes. Use of a surface coil over the axilla with supine positioning was endorsed. External rotation of the arm improved tendon visualization in some cases. When comparison was desired, an independent view of each side was preferred to a single, wide field-of-view study.[27] One group[27] recommended axial sequences including fast spin echo, another[28] recommended short-tau inversion recovery (STIR) and fat-suppressed T2, and a third[5] recommended T2. Oblique coronal fast spin echo was heavily favored by one study for grading severity of partial tears.[27]

In March 1999, Connell and colleagues[27] provided the first and only report supporting gradation of partial tear severity with MRI. MRI findings in 15 cases at a mean

5 months after injury, with 9 surgical correlations, were reviewed. In each case, MRI interpretation independently graded clavicular and sternocostal head involvement as complete, high-grade partial (>70%), moderate partial (30%–70%), and low-grade partial (<30%). Surgical findings correlated with preoperative MRI in all 9 cases (2 complete, 7 high-grade partial tears with multiple patterns). Periosteal stripping on MRI correlated with a confirmed insertional injury in 8 of 8 cases, and was considered a key finding.

In February 2000, Carrino and colleagues[28] performed a review of MRI in 10 patients with PM injuries, 6 of which had available surgical correlation, and reported 100% correlation in 5 complete and 1 partial tear. These investigators recommended the use of axial fluid-sensitive series such as STIR or fat-suppressed T2 images with small field of view and surface coils. If comparison with the contralateral side is desired, they recommend independent imaging of each. Moreover, they noted an inability to distinguish between anterior and posterior tendon laminae.

In May 2000, Lee and colleagues[5] published a descriptive and correlative study of 6 healthy subjects, 6 cadavers with gadolinium markers placed by orthopedic surgeons, and 5 clinical cases with surgical corollaries. All MRI scans for clinical cases were performed 1 to 2 weeks after injury, and findings of 3 complete and 2 partial tears correlated with surgical findings. The investigators described the use of landmarks for identifying the superior edge of the humeral insertion, which was located 1 to 1.5 cm distal to the quadrilateral space and 5 to 10 mm superior to the lateral head of the triceps.

In 2006, Zvijac and colleagues[29] reported on the impact of MRI on planned clinical management in a series of 27 patients over 5 years, and also presented the second series supporting the use of MRI to grade partial tears. All 27 patients initially underwent clinical evaluation at a mean of 3 months after injury, and a plan was established based on clinical impression of tear severity (complete, high-grade partial [>50%], or low-grade partial [<50%]) and location (intramuscular or distal; ie, musculotendinous junction to insertion). An MRI scan was subsequently obtained and evaluated by the surgeon and musculoskeletal trained radiologist. When complete or high-grade tears were diagnosed on clinical evaluation and MRI, surgery was performed. When low-grade or proximal tears were diagnosed by clinical evaluation and MRI, conservative treatment was undertaken. In 19 of 27 cases, clinical evaluation and MRI concurred. In the remaining 8 cases, MRI results were used to guide treatment. In 5 cases, tear classification was downgraded from complete to high-grade partial and the patient still proceeded to surgery. In 3 cases, diagnosis was downgraded from complete or high-grade partial tear to low-grade partial tear. At follow-up, all 3 of these patients denied stiffness, pain, deformity, or weakness, and were satisfied with treatment result. One surgically treated chronic (1-year) tear patient and 1 nonoperatively managed patient reported stiffness, pain, deformity, weakness, and dissatisfaction with their results. In both cases the clinical examination and MRI had indicated the same treatment plan. The investigators concluded that MRI may prevent unnecessary surgery in 16% (3 of 19) of cases indicated for surgery based on clinical examination alone, and that clinical examination is likely to overestimate the severity of the tear and frequently diagnose a tear location distal to the actual site of injury.

TREATMENT OPTIONS
Nonoperative Management

Nonoperative treatment is generally recommended for contusions, partial tears, muscle belly ruptures, and complete tears for lower-demand or sedentary individuals.

Studies have reported good functional recovery in activities of daily living with these injury patterns.[3,30–32] However, patients are often left with cosmetic defects or significant strength deficits that prevent full return to preinjury athletic levels.[14,18,33]

Initial nonoperative treatment involves rest, ice, control of hematoma, analgesics, and sling immobilization in the adducted and internally rotated position.[13,18] Passive and active range of motion exercises should begin within the first 2 weeks with a gradual increase to full motion over the next 6 weeks. Light resistive exercises can start at 6 to 8 weeks with gradual increases over the next 4 to 6 weeks. By 3 to 4 months, patients can resume nearly full resistance training.[13,34] Return to contact sports should be delayed for 5 to 6 months until full motion and strength return.[34] In some cases, patients should permanently avoid high-weight, low-repetition bench pressing.[35,36] Late surgical repair or reconstruction may be considered if the patient fails to progress over the first 3 to 4 months.

Operative Management

Although the PM is not required for most activities of daily living,[18,32,37] it is generally accepted that surgical repair provides the best outcomes in satisfaction, strength, cosmesis, and return to sport for young, active athletes.[3,11,14,15,18,21,30,33,36,38–41] Complete tears, including isolated sternal head/posterior lamina tears,[16] located at the myotendinous junction, intratendinous, or tendon insertion, should be repaired. A timely and accurate diagnosis of a complete tear may be delayed because of initial swelling, pain, and ecchymosis. Some investigators recommend advanced imaging to facilitate an early diagnosis for surgical repair.[5,22,24,27–29]

Surgical Techniques

Both beach-chair and supine positions through a deltopectoral or anterior axillary approach can be used.[13] Tendon to tendon, bone trough, suture anchors, and cortical buttons are commonly described techniques to repair the PM tendon. All techniques require meticulous attention to protect the long head of biceps just medial to the pectoralis tendon insertion. For intratendinous tears, direct suturing of the tendon ends may be performed if enough healthy tissue remains attached to the insertion.[12,42]

The bone trough technique (**Fig. 4**) involves creating a 5-cm vertical trough over the footprint just lateral to the bicipital groove. Four 2-mm drill holes are made 1 cm lateral to the trough. Three high-strength nonabsorbable sutures are placed in the tendon in a locking configuration. Sutures are passed into the trough, out of the drill holes, and tied over the bone bridge.[33]

The suture anchor technique (**Fig. 5**) involves removing soft tissue and lightly abrading the footprint. Two or 3 rotator cuff–sized suture anchors with 1 or 2 preloaded high-strength nonabsorbable sutures are placed in the footprint. One limb of each suture is placed in a locking fashion in the tendon. After one limb from each suture is passed through the tendon, each passed limb is tied to its free limb.[43]

The cortical button technique (**Fig. 6**) involves the same footprint preparation as for the suture anchor technique. The Pec Button (Arthrex, Naples, FL, USA) is a 2.6 × 10.9 mm titanium button that can be preloaded with 1 or 2 high-strength nonabsorbable sutures. Three 3.2-mm unicortical drill holes are made evenly spaced throughout the footprint, preferably with at least a 1-cm intervening bone bridge. The Pec Button's 45° design facilitates flipping once it contacts the far cortex, which allows unicortical engagement of the near cortex. After all of the buttons are placed, one limb from each suture is placed through the tendon and tied to its free limb, similar to the suture anchor technique.[8] Uchiyama and colleagues[44] described a similar technique using bicortical fixation with Endobuttons (Acufex; Smith & Nephew, Andover, MA, USA).

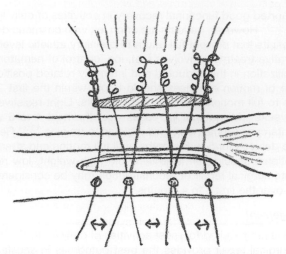

Fig. 4. Bone trough technique. A 5-cm bone trough is created lateral to the biceps tendon at the PM insertion site. Four evenly spaced 2-mm drill holes are made 1 cm lateral to the bone trough. Sutures are placed in the tendon in a locking configuration and passed into the trough, out of the drill holes, and tied over the bone bridge. (*Adapted from* Rabuck SJ, Lynch JL, Guo X, et al. Biomechanical comparison of 3 methods to repair pectoralis major ruptures. Am J Sports Med 2012;40:1635–40; with permission.)

Several recent cadaveric studies have evaluated the biomechanical comparison of the aforementioned techniques. Hart and colleagues[45] found no difference between bone trough and suture anchor techniques, with an ultimate failure load of 611 N for bone trough repair and 620 N for suture anchor repair. Mode of failure between groups

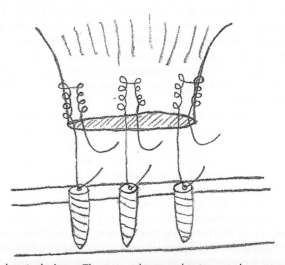

Fig. 5. Suture anchor technique. Three evenly spaced suture anchors are placed in the PM insertion site. One limb of each suture is passed in a locking fashion in the tendon and tied to its free limb. (*Adapted from* Rabuck SJ, Lynch JL, Guo X, et al. Biomechanical comparison of 3 methods to repair pectoralis major ruptures. Am J Sports Med 2012;40:1635–40; with permission.)

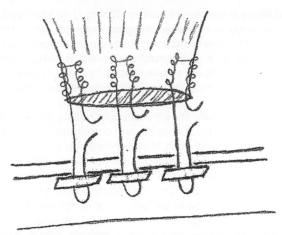

Fig. 6. Cortical button technique. Three evenly spaced cortical buttons, preloaded with high-strength nonabsorbable sutures, are placed in the PM insertion site. One limb of each suture is passed in a locking fashion in the tendon and tied to its free limb. (*Adapted from* Rabuck SJ, Lynch JL, Guo X, et al. Biomechanical comparison of 3 methods to repair pectoralis major ruptures. Am J Sports Med 2012;40:1635–40; with permission.)

did not differ, with fracture occurring in half of the bone trough group and suture breakage occurring in the entire suture anchor group. Fracture as a failure method may have been related to the higher mean age of the cadavers used (85 years). Rabuck and colleagues demonstrated,[43] in 29 cadavers with a mean age of 54.4 years, that bone trough repair showed a significantly higher load to failure compared with suture anchor repair. There was no significant difference between bone trough and cortical button or cortical button and suture anchor repair. The mean load to failure was 596 N for the bone trough group with suture breakage in 9 specimens and fracture in 1 specimen (the lowest bone mineral density specimen in the trough group). The cortical button group failed at 494 N, with suture breakage in all 10 repairs. The suture anchor group failed at 383 N, with failure occurring at the suture eyelet in 5 specimens and suture breakage in 4 specimens. Sherman and colleagues[8] compared 4 groups of 6 cadaveric specimens under intact, Pec Button repair, suture anchor repair, and transosseous suture conditions. These investigators found that intact specimens had significantly greater maximal load (1455 N) and were significantly stiffer than all 3 repair constructs. There was no significant difference in load to failure (bone trough 359 N; cortical button 353 N; suture anchor 292 N), elongation, linear stiffness, initial excursion, cyclic elongation, or footprint restoration among the 3 repair groups. All 3 repair techniques failed by suture pulling through the tendon. The pectoralis button showed significantly higher elongation and initial excursion in comparison with the intact condition.

In summary, all described techniques are effective at repairing a torn PM tendon. However, some investigators have reported that the suture anchor and cortical button techniques are easier to use because of less dissection laterally on the humerus, which the bone trough technique requires.[35]

Surgical Timing

Although there is no consensus on acute versus chronic PM injuries, a systematic review by Flint and colleagues[46] defined acute injuries as those up to 6 weeks and chronic injuries as those longer than 6 weeks. Timing is an important component, as chronic injuries may require increased surgical exposure and surgical dissection because of scarring and muscle retraction.[9] Furthermore, chronic injuries may prevent a direct repair, necessitating a reconstructive procedure using autograft or allograft tissue. Although several investigators have reported good outcomes in chronic repairs (up to 13 years after injury), most of these studies are case reports or small case series.[39,41,47,48]

More recent literature generally shows that acute repairs are technically easier and lead to improved results. In 2000, Schepsis and colleagues[33] compared patients undergoing acute repair (<2 weeks) with those undergoing chronic primary repair. No significant difference was found between groups, but there was a trend favoring acute repairs for pain relief, subjective strength, isokinetic strength evaluation, and overall satisfaction. In a meta-analysis, Bak and colleagues[11] reported a significantly higher percentage of excellent outcomes in patients undergoing acute repairs (0–8 weeks) compared with chronic repairs (9–52 weeks). In 2004, Aarima and colleagues[12] reported on their own case series and a meta-analysis. Using Bak's criteria, they showed a nonsignificant trend favoring the acute repair group (<3 weeks) for their case series. Their meta-analysis showed outcomes statistically superior to those for acute repair. In 2009, Antosh and colleagues[36] reinforced these findings by demonstrating that acute repairs (<6 weeks) led to statistically better overall DASH (Disabilities of the Arm, Shoulder, and Hand) and Work Module scores in a military population. More recently, de Castro Pochini and colleagues[15] reported better results for acute repairs (<3 weeks). Therefore, acute primary repair would seem to be the preferred treatment option for PM tears.

Rehabilitation

After repair, patients are immobilized in a sling for 6 weeks. Pendulum exercises are begun in the first week, avoiding abduction and external rotation.[13,33,34] At 6 weeks, gentle passive motion can begin in all planes of motion, and periscapular and isometric strengthening exercises can be added over the next few weeks.[16] At 3 months, the patient should have near full range of motion and can begin light resistance exercises.[13,16,33] Strengthening is progressed over the next 3 months, with a return to unrestricted activity around 6 months postoperatively.[13,33] High-weight, low-repetition exercises that involve the PM, especially flat bench, should be discouraged permanently.[16]

Complications

Reported complications from PM injuries are rare. With nonoperative treatment, persistent weakness is the most common complaint especially in the young, active patient.[11,14,18,33,39–41] Cosmetic deformity, hematoma, abscess formation, and myositis ossificans are other complications reported with nonoperative treatment.[18,49,50] Operative complications are those typically encountered with any surgical procedure such as infection, hypertrophic scar, stiffness, and rerupture.[3,41,51,52] Of note, both authors have encountered a postoperative infection in active-duty patients requiring serial debridement and irrigation. De Castro Pochini and colleagues[15] reported the possibility of foreign-body reaction, which to the authors' knowledge has not been reported by others. One of the authors has experienced multiple episodes of late (>4–6 weeks postoperatively) wound dehiscence in a patient with a sterile abscess. This patient failed repetitive multimodality wound care and ultimately responded rapidly to excision of the high tensile strength suture. Based on these experiences, the authors currently advocate restricting suture placement to the minimum required to obtain secure control of the tendon. Though not reported, injury to the medial and lateral pectoral nerves is possible from aggressive mobilization of retracted tears,[13] but should be limited if surgeons remain within the recommended safe zone for dissection.[6]

Outcomes

Studies comparing nonoperative with operative treatment overwhelmingly support surgical repair. Operative management reliably restores preinjury strength and activity levels, leads to higher patient satisfaction, and provides superior cosmetic results.[3,14,15,18,30,33,39,41]

In 1972, McEntire and colleagues[30] were one of the first to report superior functional results with surgical repair over conservative treatment. In 1979, Zeman and colleagues[18] described 4 patients that had surgical repair and 5 patients treated nonoperatively. All 4 surgical patients obtained excellent results and returned to vigorous athletic activities. All 5 nonoperative patients had good results, but none returned to their preinjury activity level. In 1989, Kretzler and Richardson[41] reported on 16 surgical patients, 13 of whom regained full strength while 2 others made significant improvement, despite between 5 and 6 years from injury to surgery.

In 1992, Wolfe and colleagues[3] demonstrated in 7 surgical patients that peak torque and work production were comparable with the uninjured side, whereas the nonoperative group had marked deficits. In 2000, Schepsis and colleagues[33] retrospectively studied 17 cases of PM ruptures that involved 13 surgical patients and 4 nonoperative patients, and reported significant differences in pain, overall satisfaction, cosmesis, and all isokinetic testing parameters favoring surgical repair. During that same year, Bak and colleagues[11] reported on a meta-analysis regarding treatment outcomes for 72 patients. The functional outcome for surgical patients was significantly better than for nonoperative patients (88% vs 27%).

In 2001, Hanna and colleagues[39] evaluated 22 PM tears with 10 undergoing surgical repair and 12 treated conservatively. For the surgical group, peak torque returned to 99% and work performed returned to 97% compared with the uninjured side. For the nonoperative group, both peak torque and work performed returned to only 56%. Both differences were significant. Most recently, in 2014, de Castro Pochini and colleagues[15] reported on a prospective study involving 60 patients divided evenly between surgical repair and nonoperative treatment. Using Bak's functional criteria,[11] the investigators found excellent or good results in 90.3% of the surgical patients versus 27.6% of the nonoperative patients. Furthermore, peak torque deficits were found in 14.3% of surgical patients, compared with 41.7% of nonoperative patients.

Military Studies

To date there have been few military studies on PM injuries. White and colleagues[10] conducted a respective review over 2 years at a busy US Army installation, identifying 52 major tendon ruptures of which 7 (14%) were PM tears. Five (71%) tears occurred while bench pressing. Antosh and colleagues[36] retrospectively reviewed all PM tears over 7 years at a US Army hospital and identified 14 surgical patients, 11 of whom ruptured the PM while bench pressing. Eight patients were repaired acutely (<6 weeks), and 6 patients were repaired in a delayed (>6 weeks) manner. Patients with acute repairs had better overall DASH and Work Module scores, with a trend to returning to work sooner with less activity-related pain. In comparison with other studies, the investigators found a 30% to 40% loss of strength in surgical patients.

Arciero and Cruser[19] presented a case report on a 20-year-old cadet at the United States Military Academy who sustained a PM tear with simultaneous anterior shoulder dislocation during an incline bench press. Arthroscopy confirmed an anterior capsulolabral complex avulsion that was treated nonoperatively. The PM tear was repaired, and the patient returned to his preinjury performance level without signs of instability. Warme and Whitaker[53] reported the first case of a PM tear while rappelling in a 34-year-old soldier on active duty. The patient felt a pop while reaching behind his back to slow his descent. A bone trough technique was used for repair. Although no follow-up was reported, the investigators advocate early surgical repair for optimum results and a return to full duty in high-demand soldiers and athletes. Komurcu and colleagues[20] reported a PM tear in a 28-year-old paratrooper who became entangled in his parachute risers. The patient underwent nonoperative treatment consisting of a 6-month rehabilitation program, with near return of full strength using dynamometric assessment. The investigators mention that if the patient had not improved, they would have encouraged surgical repair. Although this is the only published case, both authors have experienced treating patients with this injury mechanism and suspect that it is underreported.

Delayed Reconstruction

In chronic PM tears, primary repair may not be possible because of muscle retraction and involution of the residual tendon. Several investigators have reported different grafts for reconstructing the PM tendon, including Achilles tendon allograft,[54,55] bone-patellar tendon autograft,[56] hamstring autograft,[57] and fascia lata allograft.[58] Alho[26] reported a medial fascia release through a second medial incision that advanced the tendon 2 cm. De Castro Pochini and colleagues[15] recommended hamstring autograft augmentation in cases with significant tendinopathy. Furthermore, they performed augmentation in all patients after 3 months from injury. Most of these studies, however, are small case series with limited objective outcomes.

Zacchilli and colleagues[54] reported Achilles tendon allograft reconstruction in 3 military patients with chronic, complete PM tears. The average delay to surgery was 22.2 months. Using Bak's criteria,[11] 1 patient reported an excellent result and 2 patients reported good results, with an average SANE (Single Assessment Numerical Evaluation) score of 79.3. All patients returned to full active-duty military service.

The Authors' Preferred Technique

Partial ruptures that primarily involve the muscle belly are treated nonoperatively, as already described. An early and accurate diagnosis may be difficult in the acute setting because of pain, swelling, and ecchymosis. As such, an MRI is typically obtained within the first week or so to better define the extent and location of injury. Patients are discouraged from performing high-weight, low-repetition bench pressing indefinitely. For complete ruptures, the authors agree with most investigators that acute surgical management (<6–8 weeks) provides better results in patient satisfaction, strength, and return to high-level activities.

The patient is placed in the modified beach-chair position under general anesthesia with full muscle paralysis. The distal part of a deltopectoral approach is used through a 6- to 7-cm incision. The nature of injury is confirmed, and high-strength traction sutures are placed in a locking manner from the tendon end to the musculotendinous junction. The tendon frequently telescopes into the muscle belly, and must be carefully dissected along its edge with scissors to expose adequate tissue for repair. The tendon and muscle belly are then mobilized by releasing adhesions through digital and blunt dissection. Circumferential release of adhesions is vital to adequately mobilize the tendon to the footprint. However, the release should not proceed more than 8 cm medially to avoid the medial and lateral pectoral nerves. The footprint is prepared by removing soft tissue and lightly decorticating the bone. Three unicortical holes are evenly drilled throughout the footprint using a 3.2-mm spade-tipped drill pin (Arthrex). It is important when placing these drill holes to maintain at least 1-cm bone bridges. However, one must also take care to keep tendon dimensions in mind. The width of the tendon decreases after a rupture. The distance between the most proximal and distal holes should not exceed the width of the ruptured tendon, or the surgeon risks excessive gap formation at the repair site. Three Pec Buttons (Arthrex) preloaded with two #2 FiberWires (Arthrex) are inserted into each drill hole, ensuring that the button flips and engages the anterior cortex. One limb from each suture is passed up and back down the tendon in a locking fashion. The last throw exits on the anterior surface, which aids in pushing the tendon to bone. The second suture from each button is passed as a horizontal mattress or Kessler stitch. The sternal head sutures are passed first using the superior and middle buttons, which places the sternal head deep and proximal to the clavicular head. Once all sutures are passed, the sternal head Krakow sutures (proximal) are tied, followed by the clavicular head sutures. The Kessler or horizontal suture limbs are then tied to reinforce contact at the footprint. The long head of the biceps tendon is protected throughout the repair to avoid injury or incorporation under the footprint. The wound is copiously irrigated and closed in layers. A shoulder immobilizer is placed, and the patient is started on the rehabilitation protocol as described earlier.

SUMMARY

PM tears most commonly occur in the young athletic male while performing weight-lifting exercises, but can result from any activity whereby the arm is maximally contracted in an extended and externally rotated position. Patients typically present with acute pain, swelling, ecchymosis, deformity, and weakness with adduction and internal rotation. Diagnosis of PM tears can usually be made by history and physical examination, but MRI can be helpful in identifying the extent and location of injury. Most tears occur near the tendon insertion. Nonoperative treatment is generally reserved for proximal tears, low-grade partial tears, and tears in sedentary patients. In most cases these patients will resume full activities of daily living. For all other tears, especially in the young, active athlete, acute (<6 weeks) repair is recommended to return the patient to full strength and function.

REFERENCES

1. Fung L, Wong B, Ravichandiran K, et al. Three-dimensional study of pectoralis major muscle and tendon architecture. Clin Anat 2009;22:500–8. http://dx.doi.org/10.1002/ca.20784.
2. Porzionato A, Mcchi V, Stecco C, et al. Surgical anatomy of the pectoral nerves and the pectoral musculature. Clin Anat 2012;25:559–75.
3. Wolfe SW, Wickiewicz TL, Cavanaugh JT. Ruptures of the pectoralis major muscle: an anatomic and clinical analysis. Am J Sports Med 1992;20:587–93. http://dx.doi.org/10.1177/036354659202000517.
4. Tobin GR. Pectoralis major segmental anatomy and segmentally split pectoralis major flaps. Plast Reconstr Surg 1985;75:814–24.
5. Lee J, Brookenthal KR, Ramsey ML, et al. MR imaging assessment of the pectoralis major myotendinous unit: an MR imaging-anatomic correlative study with surgical correlation. Am J Roentgenol 2000;174:1371–5.

6. Klepps SJ, Goldfarb C, Flatow E, et al. Anatomic evaluation of the subcoracoid pectoralis major transfer in human cadavers. J Shoulder Elbow Surg 2001;10: 453–9.

7. Carey P, Owens BD. Insertional footprint anatomy of the pectoralis major tendon. Orthopedics 2010;33(1):23. http://dx.doi.org/10.3928/01477447-20091124-27.

8. Sherman SL, Lin EC, Verma NN, et al. Biomechanical analysis of the pectoralis major tendon and comparison of techniques for tendo-osseous repair. Am J Sports Med 2012;40:1887–94. http://dx.doi.org/10.1177/0363546512452849.

9. ElMaraghy AW, Devereaux MW. A systematic review and comprehensive classification of pectoralis major tears. J Shoulder Elbow Surg 2012;21:412–22.

10. White DW, Wenke JC, Mosely DS, et al. Incidence of major tendon ruptures and anterior cruciate ligament tears in US Army soldiers. Am J Sports Med 2007;35: 1308–14. http://dx.doi.org/10.1177/0363546507301256.

11. Bak K, Cameron EA, Henderson IJ. Rupture of the pectoralis major: a meta-analysis of 112 cases. Knee Surg Sports Traumatol Arthrosc 2000;8:113–9. http://dx.doi. org/10.1007/s001670050197.

12. Aarima V, Rantanen J, Heikkila J, et al. Rupture of the pectoralis major muscle. Am J Sports Med 2004;32:1256–62. http://dx.doi.org/10.1177/0363546503261137.

13. Provencher MT, Handfield K, Boniquit NT, et al. Injuries to the pectoralis major muscle: diagnosis and management. Am J Sports Med 2010;38:1693–705. http://dx.doi.org/10.1177/0363546509348051.

14. de Castro Pochini A, Ejnisman B, Andreoli CV, et al. Pectoralis major muscle ruptures in athletes: a prospective study. Am J Sports Med 2010;38:92–8. http://dx. doi.org/10.1177/0363546509347995.

15. de Castro Pochini A, Andreoli CV, Belangero PS, et al. Clinical considerations for the surgical treatment of pectoralis major muscle ruptures based on 60 cases: a prospective study and literature. Am J Sports Med 2014;42:95–102. http://dx. doi.org/10.1177/0363546513506556.

16. Petilon J, Carr DR, Sekiya JK, et al. Pectoralis major muscle injuries: evaluation and management. J Am Acad Orthop Surg 2005;13:59–68.

17. Tietjen R. Closed injuries of the pectoralis major muscle. J Trauma 1980;20: 262–4.

18. Zeman SC, Rosenfeld RT, Lipscomb PR. Tears of the pectoralis major muscle. Am J Sports Med 1979;7:343–7.

19. Arciero RA, Cruser DL. Pectoralis major rupture with simultaneous anterior dislocation of the shoulder. J Shoulder Elbow Surg 1997;6:318–20.

20. Komurcu M, Yildiz Y, Ozdemir MT, et al. Rupture of the pectoralis major muscle in a paratrooper. Aviat Space Environ Med 2004;75:81–4.

21. Pavlik A, Csépai D, Berkes I. Surgical treatment of pectoralis major rupture in athletes. Knee Surg Sports Traumatol Arthrosc 1998;6:129–33.

22. Weaver JS, Jacobson JA, Jamadar DA, et al. Sonographic findings of pectoralis major tears with surgical, clinical, and magnetic resonance imaging correlation in 6 patients. J Ultrasound Med 2005;24:25–31.

23. Lee SJ, Jacobson JA, Kim SM, et al. Distal pectoralis major tears: sonographic characterization and potential diagnostic pitfalls. J Ultrasound Med 2013;32: 2075–81. http://dx.doi.org/10.7863/ultra.32.12.2075.

24. Miller MD, Johnson DL, Fu FH, et al. Rupture of the pectoralis major muscle in a collegiate football player. Use of magnetic resonance imaging in early diagnosis. Am J Sports Med 1993;21:475–7.

25. Ohashi K, El-Khoury GY, Albright JP, et al. MRI of complete rupture of the pectoralis major muscle. Skeletal Radiol 1996;25:625–8.

26. Alho A. Ruptured pectoralis major tendon. A case report on delayed repair with muscle advancement. Acta Orthop Scand 1994;65:652–3.
27. Connell DA, Potter HG, Sherman MF, et al. Injuries of the pectoralis major muscle: evaluation with MR imaging. Radiology 1999;210:785–91.
28. Carrino JA, Chandnanni VP, Mitchell DB, et al. Pectoralis major muscle and tendon tears: diagnosis and grading using magnetic resonance imaging. Skeletal Radiol 2000;29:305–13.
29. Zvijac JE, Schurhoff MR, Hechtman KS, et al. Pectoralis major tears: correlation of magnetic resonance imaging and treatment strategies. Am J Sports Med 2006;34:289–94.
30. McEntire JE, Hess WE, Coleman SS. Rupture of the pectoralis major muscle. A report of eleven injuries and review of fifty-six. J Bone Joint Surg Am 1972;54:1040–6.
31. Scott BW, Wallace WA, Barton MA. Diagnosis and assessment of pectoralis major rupture by dynamometry. J Bone Joint Surg Br 1992;74:111–3.
32. Beloosesky Y, Grinblat J, Weiss A, et al. Pectoralis major rupture in elderly patients: a clinical study of 13 patients. Clin Orthop Relat Res 2003;413:164–9.
33. Schepsis AA, Grafe MW, Jones HP, et al. Rupture of the pectoralis major: outcome after repair of acute and chronic injuries. Am J Sports Med 2000;28:9–15.
34. Potter BK, Lehman RA Jr, Doukas WC. Pectoralis major ruptures. Am J Orthop (Belle Mead NJ) 2006;35:189–95.
35. Elkhousy H. Chapter 17, Section G. In: DeLee JC, Drez DD, Miller MD, editors. DeLee & Drez's orthopaedic sports medicine, vol. 1, 3rd edition. Philadelphia: Saunders Elsevier; 2010. p. 900–7.
36. Antosh IJ, Grassbaugh JA, Parada SA, et al. Pectoralis major tendon repairs in the active-duty population. Am J Orthop 2009;38:26–30.
37. Marmor I, Bechtol C, Hall C. Pectoralis major muscle. J Bone Joint Surg Am 1961;43:81–7.
38. Quinlan JF, Molloy M, Hurson BJ. Pectoralis major tendon ruptures: when to operate. Br J Sports Med 2002;36:226–8. http://dx.doi.org/10.1136/bjsm.36.3.226.
39. Hanna CM, Glenny AB, Stanley SN, et al. Pectoralis major tears: comparison of surgical and conservative treatment. Br J Sports Med 2001;35(3):202. http://dx.doi.org/10.1136/bjsm.35.3.202.
40. Park JY, Espiniella JL. Rupture of pectoralis major muscle. A case report and review of literature. J Bone Joint Surg Am 1970;52:577–81.
41. Kretzler HH, Richardson AB. Rupture of the pectoralis major muscle. Am J Sports Med 1989;17:453–8.
42. Dodds SD, Wolfe SW. Injuries to the pectoralis major. Sports Med 2002;32:945–52.
43. Rabuck SJ, Lynch JL, Guo X, et al. Biomechanical comparison of 3 methods to repair pectoralis major ruptures. Am J Sports Med 2012;40:1635–40. http://dx.doi.org/10.1177/0363546512449291.
44. Uchiyama Y, Miyazaki S, Tamaki T, et al. Clinical results of a surgical technique using endobuttons for complete tendon tear of pectoralis major muscle: report of five cases. Sports Med Arthrosc Rehabil Ther Technol 2011;28:20. http://dx.doi.org/10.1186/1758-2555-3-20.
45. Hart ND, Lindsey DP, McAdams TR. Pectoralis major tendon rupture: a biomechanical analysis of repair techniques. J Orthop Res 2011;29:1783–7. http://dx.doi.org/10.1002/jor.21438.
46. Flint JH, Wade AM, Giuliani J, et al. Defining the terms acute and chronic in orthopaedic sports injuries: a systematic review. Am J Sports Med 2014;42:235–41. http://dx.doi.org/10.1177/0363546513490656.

47. Anbari A, Kelly JD, Moyer RA. Delayed repair of a ruptured pectoralis major muscle: a case report. Am J Sports Med 2000;28:254–6.
48. Lindebaum BL. Delayed repair of a ruptured pectoralis major muscle. Clin orthop 1975;109:120–1.
49. Purnell R. Rupture of the pectoralis major: a complication. Injury 1988;19:284.
50. Patissier P. Malaides des bouchers. Traite des maladies des artisans. Paris: Chez J-B Baillere Libraire; 1822. p. 162–5.
51. Kakwani RG, Matthews JJ, Kumar KM, et al. Rupture of the pectoralis major muscle: surgical treatment in athletes. Int Orthop 2007;31:159–63.
52. Pai VS, Simison AJ. A rare complication of pectoralis major rupture. Aust N Z J Surg 1995;65:694–5.
53. Warme WJ, Whitaker DC. Pectoralis major tendon avulsion from rappelling. Mil Med 2004;169:151–4.
54. Zacchilli MA, Fowler JT, Owens BD. Allograft reconstruction of chronic pectoralis major tendon ruptures. J Surg Orthop Adv 2013;22(1):95–102. http://dx.doi.org/10.3113/JSOA.2013.0095.
55. Joseph TA, DeFranco MJ, Weiker GG. Delayed repair of a pectoralis major tendon rupture with allograft: a case report. J Shoulder Elbow Surg 2003;12(1):101–4. http://dx.doi.org/10.1067/mse.2003.128200.
56. Zafra M, Muñoz F, Carpintero P. Chronic rupture of the pectoralis major muscle: report of two cases. Acta Orthop Belg 2005;71(1):107–10.
57. Schachter AK, White BJ, Namkoong S, et al. Revision reconstruction of a pectoralis major tendon rupture using hamstring autograft: a case report. Am J Sports Med 2006;34(2):295–8. http://dx.doi.org/10.1177/0363546505278697.
58. Sikka RS, Neault M, Guanche CA. Reconstruction of the pectoralis major tendon with fascia lata allograft. Orthopedics 2005;28(10):1199–201.

Snapping Scapula Syndrome in the Military

Jeanne C. Patzkowski, MD[a],*, Brett D. Owens, MD[b], Travis C. Burns, MD[a]

KEYWORDS

- Snapping scapula syndrome • Chest wall • Military • Bursa

KEY POINTS

- Snapping scapula syndrome is caused by abnormal interaction between the scapula and chest wall and may be caused by an osseous or soft tissue mass, abnormal muscle dynamics, or chronic scapulothoracic bursitis.
- Snapping scapula syndrome may be more prevalent in the military because of physical fitness standards requiring intense upper body exercise, prolonged heavy load bearing through the shoulder girdle, and use of protective gear that applies nonphysiologic forces to the scapulothoracic articulation.
- Initial treatment is nonoperative. Corticosteroid injections into inflamed bursae may be diagnostic and therapeutic.
- Arthroscopic bursectomy with partial scapulectomy may help patients who are refractory to nonoperative measures.
- Anatomy of the scapulothoracic articulation is complex and arthroscopy should only be attempted after obtaining a thorough understanding of this region.

INTRODUCTION: NATURE OF THE PROBLEM

The scapulothoracic joint is a complex, noncongruent articulation between the scapula and the chest wall. Motion and stability of the scapula are controlled through the dynamic interaction of the surrounding musculature. The scapula is a triangular bone with 3 borders (medial, lateral, and superior) and 3 angles (superomedial, inferomedial, and lateral), and the costal surface is concave to match the convexity of the chest wall.[1–3] The acuity of the superomedial angle varies widely, ranging between 124° and 162° relative to the scapular body.[4] Two bursae, the infraserratus and supraserratus, are consistently found in this region. The infraserratus bursa lies between the

Disclosure: The views expressed in this article are those of the authors only and do not represent the views of the San Antonio Military Medical Center, Keller Army Community Hospital, the United States Army or Department of Defense.
[a] Orthopaedic Surgery Service, San Antonio Military Medical Center, 3851 Roger Brooke Drive, Fort Sam Houston, TX 78234, USA; [b] Orthopaedic Surgery Service, Keller Army Community Hospital, 900 Washington Road, West Point, NY 10996, USA
* Corresponding author.
E-mail address: jeanne.patzkowski@gmail.com

Clin Sports Med 33 (2014) 757–766
http://dx.doi.org/10.1016/j.csm.2014.06.003
0278-5919/14/$ – see front matter Published by Elsevier Inc.

sportsmed.theclinics.com

serratus anterior muscle and the chest wall, whereas the supraserratus bursa is found between the serratus anterior and subscapularis musculature.[2] Additional minor bursae are variably noted and are considered pathologic. They are typically located at the superomedial angle, inferomedial angle, and at the medial base of the spine of the scapula underneath the trapezius (trapezoid bursa).[2]

Several neurovascular structures lie in the vicinity of the scapula (**Fig. 1**). The spinal accessory nerve travels on the deep surface of the trapezius and enters the interval between the superomedial scapula and the trapezius lateral to the fibers of the levator scapulae. It crosses the superior border of the scapula approximately 3 cm lateral to the superomedial angle and terminates in the body of the trapezius.[5] A superficial branch of the transverse cervical artery runs alongside the spinal accessory nerve. The dorsal scapular artery and nerve travel approximately 1 cm medial to the medial border of the scapula, deep to the rhomboid major and minor. The long thoracic nerve resides on the anterolateral surface of the serratus anterior and could be injured with far anterior instrumentation in the space between the subscapularis and serratus anterior. The suprascapular artery and nerve run along the superior border of the scapula toward the suprascapular notch.[6,7]

Snapping scapula syndrome may be the result of osseous or soft tissue masses within the scapulothoracic space. Anatomic causes include osseous masses such as osteochondroma, or rarely chondrosarcoma in older patients, elastofibroma, abnormal scapular anatomy (ex. a superomedial scapular angle less than 140 yielding excessive anterior angulation and contact with the rib cage), fibrotic or anomalous muscle, and malunion of scapula or rib fractures.[1–3,8,9] Scapulothoracic bursitis may also be involved in the pathophysiology of snapping scapula syndrome and is likely the result of inflammation related to overuse of the shoulder girdle. With continued

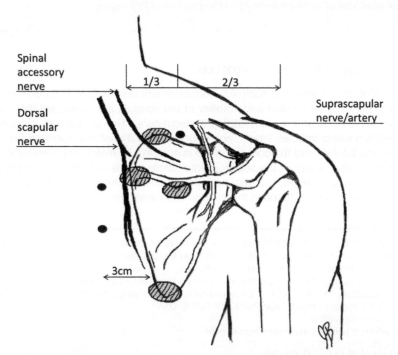

Fig. 1. Scapulothoracic anatomy. Black circles represent arthroscopic portals. Dashed ovals represent deep bursae.

irritation, fibrotic changes may take place within the various bursae leading to worsening of symptoms and overt snapping (see **Fig. 1**).[10] Postural abnormalities and excessive thoracic kyphosis may alter scapulothoracic motion as well.[11]

Symptoms in snapping scapula syndrome vary widely. Patients may complain of intermittent pain and bursitis or disabling pain and loud crepitus.[1] Pain is typically activity related and may have its onset after a traumatic injury or develop insidiously.[2,3] Symptoms are exacerbated with repetitive overhead activity or push-ups, and are typically located at the superomedial or, less commonly, the inferomedial angle.[2,3] The patient may show winging of the scapula caused by nerve or muscle injury, and there may be a palpable fullness in the setting of an underlying mass.[2]

Military service members must adhere to strict physical fitness standards in order to remain on active duty. Push-ups are among the most common exercises performed in military training and are tested in each of the services' routine physical fitness assessments. Pull-ups, obstacle courses, low crawls, and upper body weight lifting are also frequent components of service members' basic physical fitness routines. During training and deployment scenarios, service members are required to carry 35 to 55 kg (80–120 pounds) of gear for long distances, primarily using upper extremity load-bearing equipment. Although rare, winging of the scapula from nerve injury or rhomboid and trapezius muscle rupture has been reported secondary to backpack use,[12] highlighting the significant burden applied to the shoulder girdle with heavy packs. Historical reports show substantial increases in the loads borne by soldiers during combat operations, and efforts to study load distribution have been underway since the late 1980s. Multiple medical problems have been directly associated with heavy load bearing during military training, including back pain and so-called rucksack palsy. Rucksack palsy is well described and likely related to traction injury of the C5 and C6 nerve roots with symptoms ranging from numbness and cramping to scapular crepitus to permanent scapular winging.[13] In addition to the weight on the shoulder girdle, military packs and body armor plates apply nonphysiologic compressive forces to the scapulothoracic articulation, potentially contributing to malposition, bursitis, and crepitus.

Imaging modalities are an important part of the work-up for snapping scapula syndrome, particularly to rule out bony or soft tissue masses that may be the underlying cause of the pain or crepitus. Plain radiographs consisting of shoulder anteroposterior, lateral scapular, and axillary views are obtained (**Fig. 2**). Computed tomography (CT) or magnetic resonance imaging (MRI) of the scapulothoracic articulation may be helpful when physical examination or radiographs raise suspicion for a soft tissue or osseous mass. Three-dimensional CT scanning may be more sensitive than plain radiography and conventional CT for detecting subtle anatomic variations in those patients who fail to respond to conservative management.[14] However, many patients have no identifiable anatomic cause for their symptoms.

Initial management is primarily nonoperative, consisting of activity modification, antiinflammatory medication, and physical therapy. Physical therapy is directed at stretching and strengthening of periscapular musculature, restoring thoracic extension, and postural corrections.[15,16] Corticosteroid injections into inflamed bursae may assist with diagnosis and provide symptomatic relief.[10,15]

For those patients whose symptoms are refractory to nonoperative management, surgery may be beneficial. Surgery is primarily designed to remove the inflamed bursae with partial scapulectomy, which can be performed through open, arthroscopic, or combined techniques. Arthroscopic bursectomy with partial scapulectomy typically requires less dissection of the periscapular musculature and results in quicker rehabilitation.[7,17–22]

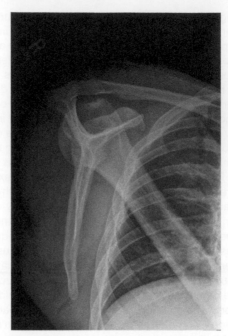

Fig. 2. Lateral scapula radiograph.

INDICATIONS/CONTRAINDICATIONS

Indications:

- Symptomatic snapping scapula/scapulothoracic bursitis
- Persistent pain and disability after appropriate nonoperative therapy and activity restrictions

Contraindications:

- Nerve palsy
- Periscapular muscle wasting
- Thoracic kyphosis
- Voluntary snapping (relative)
- No relief with local anesthetic injection into symptomatic bursa (relative)
- Cervical spine disease (relative)

SURGICAL TECHNIQUE/PROCEDURE

During preoperative planning it is imperative to ensure that the patient's history and physical examination are consistent with a diagnosis of snapping scapula syndrome or scapulothoracic bursitis. Obtain good quality plain films and CT scan or MRI if there is suspicion for a space-occupying lesion requiring further characterization. If there are any suspected neurologic abnormalities, consider cervical spine imaging or electromyographic studies as indicated.

During surgery, patients may be positioned prone or in the lateral decubitus position. If concomitant glenohumeral arthroscopy is planned, the lateral position is preferred. Anesthesia is typically general with or without the use of a regional nerve block. The arm is placed into the chicken-wing position of shoulder extension and internal rotation (**Fig. 3**). Table position in 10° to 15° of reverse Trendelenburg may help avoid extravasation of arthroscopy fluid into the neck.

For complete visualization of the scapulothoracic space both the 30° and 70° arthroscope are recommended. A standard 4.5-mm shaver and radiofrequency ablation device should be sufficient for bursectomy. We recommend the 5.5-mm burr for partial scapulectomy.

Before establishing the portals, mark out the superomedial angle of the scapula, lateral acromion, spine of scapula, inferomedial angle, and medial (vertebral) border. Place mark at the junction of the medial and middle thirds on a line between the superomedial angle of the scapula and the lateral border of the acromion (location of the superior portal). Establish the medial portal 2 to 3 cm medial to the medial border of the scapula at or below the level of the scapular spine (**Fig. 4**). Establish a second medial portal inferior to the initial portal if bursectomy is required at the inferomedial angle. The inferior portal can also serve as the viewing portal with the more superior portal used for instrumentation while working on the superomedial angle.

With the arm in the chicken-wing position place the arthroscopic cannula with trocar in the scapulothoracic space with care to direct the blunt cannula parallel to the chest wall. Create the superior portal with an inside-out technique. With the trochar in the superior of the 2 medial portals, direct the trocar superiorly and laterally, aiming for the mark at the junction of the middle one-third and lateral two-thirds of the line between the superomedial angle and lateral acromion.[7] Incise over the palpable tip of the blunt trocar to create the portal (**Fig. 5**).

Remove soft tissue and inflamed bursa from the undersurface of the superomedial corner using radiofrequency wand or shaver, similar to the technique for subacromial bursectomy (**Figs. 6 and 7**). Insert an 18-gauge needle into the medial aspect of scapula 1 cm superior to the scapular spine to mark the medialmost extent of your scapular resection (**Fig. 8**). This technique protects the dorsal scapular nerve and artery, which are located approximately 1 cm medial to the medial border of the scapula.[6] Using the burr, resect bone from the superomedial corner. Medial resection should be limited to the level of the medial needle and lateral resection should be limited to a line connecting the superior portal to a point centered between the inferior pole and the scapular spine (**Figs. 9 and 10**).[18]

The amount of bony resection necessary at the superomedial angle is controversial. Most investigators recommend 2 to 3 cm from the superomedial corner if an obvious

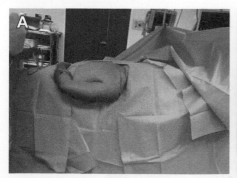
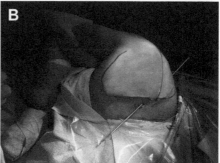

Fig. 3. (*A*) Chicken-wing position for arthroscopy (prone). (*B*) Chicken-wing position for arthroscopy (lateral decubitus).

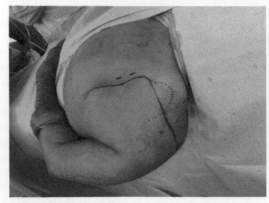

Fig. 4. Mark superior and medial portals.

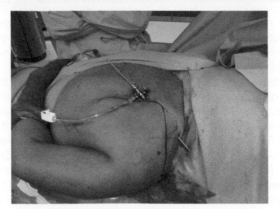

Fig. 5. Create superior portal with inside-out technique.

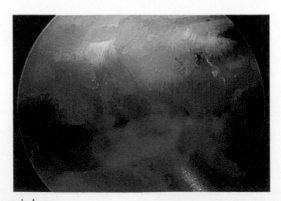

Fig. 6. Scapulothoracic bursa.

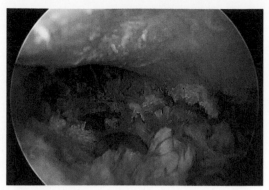
Fig. 7. Completed scapulothoracic bursectomy.

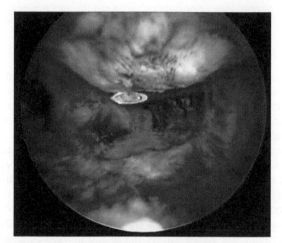
Fig. 8. Needle localization of superomedial angle of scapula.

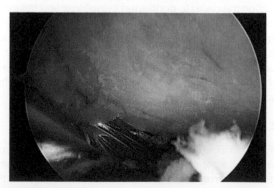
Fig. 9. Superomedial angle of scapula.

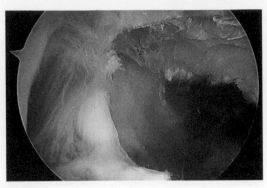

Fig. 10. Completed resection.

osseous prominence is not visualized.[18,22] Remember that the findings may be altered secondary to soft tissue distortion from arthroscopy fluid. Portals are closed in a standard fashion with absorbable or nonabsorbable suture and a simple internal rotation sling is applied.

COMPLICATIONS AND MANAGEMENT

Chest wall penetration is the most serious complication, but is easily prevented with appropriate technique. Keeping the arm in the chicken-wing position elevates the scapula away from the chest wall and facilitates instrument insertion. When entering the scapulothoracic space, always direct the instruments parallel to the chest wall to avoid chest wall penetration.

Multiple neurovascular structures are adjacent to the scapula and at risk during scapulothoracic arthroscopy. In particular, the dorsal scapular nerve and artery and spinal accessory nerve traverse adjacent to the medial border of the scapula. They can be protected by placing the medial portals 2 to 3 cm medial to the medial border of the scapula and below the level of the scapular spine.[6] Avoid use of the shaver or radiofrequency wand medial to the medial border to avoid drawing the structures into the field. The suprascapular nerve travels under the transverse scapular ligament in the suprascapular notch, with the artery traveling above the ligament. These structures are protected by placing the superior portal at the junction of the middle and medial thirds of a line connecting the superomedial border of the scapula to the lateral acromion and limiting lateral bony resection to the previously described safe zone.

Inadequate resection may lead to continued symptoms and failure of the procedure. The proper amount of bony resection is controversial. Performing an examination under anesthesia after resection to ensure no residual crepitus or impingement may help avoid this complication. Excessive resection may be prevented by placing needles at bony landmarks because arthroscopic localization may be challenging. Intraoperative fluoroscopy may help verify landmarks and extent of resection, although its use has not been well described.

POSTOPERATIVE CARE

Patients are initially immobilized in a sling for comfort. They may discontinue use of the sling within the first week after surgery. Pendulum exercises and passive motion are initiated immediately with progression to active motion and strengthening exercises to tolerance. As patients regain motion, they are referred to supervised physical therapy to assist with thoracic extension/posture training and periscapular muscle strengthening.

OUTCOMES

Most reported outcomes are from small retrospective case series. Pearse and colleagues[20] evaluated 13 patients, 10 of whom underwent bursectomy alone, and an additional 3 who had resection of the superomedial angle. Nine reported improvement in their symptoms, 6 were pain free, and 3 reported moderate pain. Eight of 9 patients returned to work and 6 returned to presymptomatic sporting activities. Millett and colleagues[19] evaluated 21 shoulders undergoing scapulothoracic bursectomy alone (2) or bursectomy with partial scapulectomy (19). The overall group had a significant improvement in American Shoulder and Elbow Surgeon (ASES) scores (average score of 53 before surgery improving to 73 after surgery), visual analog scale (VAS) (9 before surgery to 5 after surgery), QuickDASH (shortened version of Disabilities of Arm, and Hand) and Single Assessment Numeric Evaluation (SANE) scores. Younger patients and those who had bursectomy alone were noted to have smaller improvements in ASES scores and to be less satisfied overall with their care. Three (13%) required revision for persistent pain and crepitus. Pavlik and colleagues[17] reported on 10 patients undergoing arthroscopic bursectomy with partial scapulectomy and noted complete resolution of symptoms in 2 patients, decreased symptoms in 8, and subjective good/excellent results in 9. Only 1 patient reported that residual symptoms were bothersome. Nine of 10 returned to work and 6 of 9 returned to previous sporting activity. Each report emphasizes the importance of proper patient selection, and shows that good results do not necessarily imply complete resolution of symptoms.

SUMMARY

Snapping scapula syndrome is a rare condition resulting in painful crepitus of the scapulothoracic articulation that may be more common in a military population because of significant upper extremity load-bearing activities. Conservative management is the first-line therapy and is successful in up to 80% of patients. For those patients who fail conservative management, arthroscopic bursectomy and partial scapulectomy is a reasonable option, but is technically demanding and requires an in-depth understanding of the complex anatomy of the scapulothoracic region.

REFERENCES

1. Gaskill T, Millett PJ. Snapping scapula syndrome: diagnosis and management. J Am Acad Orthop Surg 2013;21:214–24.
2. Kuhne M, Boniquit N, Ghodadra N, et al. The snapping scapula: diagnosis and treatment. Arthroscopy 2009;25:1298–311.
3. Lazar MA, Kwon YW, Rokito AS. Snapping scapula syndrome. J Bone Joint Surg Am 2009;91:2251–62.
4. Aggarwal A, Wahee P, Harjeet, et al. Variable osseous anatomy of costal surface of scapula and its implications in relation to snapping scapula syndrome. Surg Radiol Anat 2011;33:135–40.
5. Williams GR, Shakil M, Klimkiewicz J, et al. Anatomy of the scapulothoracic articulation. Clin Orthop Relat Res 1999;359:237–46.
6. Ruland LJ, Ruland CM, Mathews LS. Scapulothoracic anatomy for the arthroscopist. Arthroscopy 1995;11:52–6.

7. Chan B, Chakrabarti AJ, Bell SN. An alternative portal for scapulothoracic arthroscopy. J Shoulder Elbow Surg 2002;11:235–8.

8. Edelson JG. Variations in the anatomy of the scapula with reference to the snapping scapula. Clin Orthop Relat Res 1996;322:111–5.

9. Totlis T, Konstantinidis GA, Karanassos MT, et al. Bony structures related to snapping scapula: correlation to gender, side and age. Surg Radiol Anat 2013;36(1):3–9.

10. Kuhn JE, Plancher KD, Hawkins RJ. Symptomatic scapulothoracic crepitus and bursitis. J Am Acad Orthop Surg 1998;6:267–73.

11. Kibler WB, McMullen J. Scapular dyskinesis and its relation to shoulder pain. J Am Acad Orthop Surg 2003;11:142–51.

12. Lee S, Kim J, Lee S, et al. Winged scapula caused by rhomboideus and trapezius muscles rupture associated with repetitive minor trauma: a case report. J Korean Med Sci 2006;214:581–4.

13. Knapick JJ, Reynolds KL, Harman E. Soldier load carriage: historical, physiological, biomechanical and medical aspects. Mil Med 2004;169:45–56.

14. Mozes G, Bickels J, Ovadia D, et al. The use of three-dimensional computed tomography in evaluating snapping scapula syndrome. Orthopedics 1999;22: 1029–33.

15. Manske RC, Reiman MP, Stovak ML. Nonoperative and operative management of snapping scapula. Am J Sports Med 2004;32:1554–65.

16. Conduah AH, Baker CL, Baker CL. Clinical management of scapulothoracic bursitis and the snapping scapula. Sports Health 2010;2:147–55.

17. Pavlik A, Ang K, Coghlan J, et al. Arthroscopic treatment of painful snapping of the scapula by using a new superior portal. Arthroscopy 2003;19:608–12.

18. Bell SN, van Riet RP. Safe zone for arthroscopic resection of the superomedial scapular border in the treatment of snapping scapula syndrome. J Shoulder Elbow Surg 2008;17:647–9.

19. Millett PJ, Gaskill TR, Horan MP, et al. Technique and outcomes of arthroscopic scapulothoracic bursectomy and partial scapulectomy. Arthroscopy 2012;28: 1776–83.

20. Pearse EO, Bruguera J, Massoud SM, et al. Arthroscopic management of the painful snapping scapula. Arthroscopy 2006;22:755–61.

21. Blond L, Rechter S. Arthroscopic treatment for snapping scapula: a prospective case series. Eur J Orthop Surg Traumatol 2013;24(2):159–64.

22. Lehtinen JT, Tetreault P, Warner JJ. Arthroscopic management of painful and stiff scapulothoracic articulation. Arthroscopy 2003;19(4):E28.

Index

Note: Page numbers of article titles are in **boldface** type.

Clin Sports Med 33 (2014) 767–771
http://dx.doi.org/10.1016/S0278-5919(14)00076-3
0278-5919/14/$ – see front matter © 2014 Elsevier Inc. All rights reserved.

sportsmed.theclinics.com

United States Postal Service

Statement of Ownership, Management, and Circulation
(All Periodicals Publications Except Requester Publications)

1. Publication Title	2. Publication Number	3. Filing Date
Clinics in Sports Medicine	0 0 0 - 7 0 2	9/14/14

4. Issue Frequency	5. Number of Issues Published Annually	6. Annual Subscription Price
Jan, Apr, Jul, Oct	4	$340.00

7. Complete Mailing Address of Known Office of Publication (Not printer) (Street, city, county, state, and ZIP+4®)

Elsevier Inc.
360 Park Avenue South
New York, NY 10010-1710

Contact Person
Stephen R. Bushing
Telephone (Include area code)
215-239-3688

8. Complete Mailing Address of Headquarters or General Business Office of Publisher (Not printer)

Elsevier Inc., 360 Park Avenue South, New York, NY 10010-1710

9. Full Names and Complete Mailing Addresses of Publisher, Editor, and Managing Editor (Do not leave blank)

Publisher (Name and complete mailing address)

Linda Belfus, Elsevier, Inc. 1600 John F. Kennedy Blvd. Suite 1800, Philadelphia, PA 19103-2899

Editor (Name and complete mailing address)

Jennifer Flynn-Briggs, Elsevier, Inc., 1600 John F. Kennedy Blvd. Suite 1800, Philadelphia, PA 19103-2899

Managing Editor (Name and complete mailing address)

Adrianne Brigido, Elsevier, Inc., 1600 John F. Kennedy Blvd. Suite 1800, Philadelphia, PA 19103-2899

10. Owner (Do not leave blank. If the publication is owned by a corporation, give the name and address of the corporation immediately followed by the names and addresses of all stockholders owning or holding 1 percent or more of the total amount of stock. If not owned by a corporation, give the names and addresses of the individual owners. If owned by a partnership or other unincorporated firm, give its name and address as well as those of each individual owner. If the publication is published by a nonprofit organization, give its name and address.)

Full Name	Complete Mailing Address
Wholly owned subsidiary of	1600 John F. Kennedy Blvd, Ste. 1800
Reed/Elsevier, US holdings	Philadelphia, PA 19103-2899

11. Known Bondholders, Mortgagees, and Other Security Holders Owning or Holding 1 Percent or More of Total Amount of Bonds, Mortgages, or Other Securities. If none, check box. ☑ None

Full Name	Complete Mailing Address
N/A	

12. Tax Status (For completion by nonprofit organizations authorized to mail at nonprofit rates) (Check one)
The purpose, function, and nonprofit status of this organization and the exempt status for federal income tax purposes:
☐ Has Not Changed During Preceding 12 Months
☐ Has Changed During Preceding 12 Months (Publisher must submit explanation of change with this statement)

PS Form 3526, August 2012 (Page 1 of 3 (Instructions Page 3)) PSN 7530-01-000-9931 PRIVACY NOTICE: See our Privacy policy in www.usps.com

---

13. Publication Title		14. Issue Date for Circulation Data Below
Surgical Pathology Clinics		July 2014

15. Extent and Nature of Circulation			14. Average No. Copies Each Issue During Preceding 12 Months	No. Copies of Single Issue Published Nearest to Filing Date
a. Total Number of Copies (Net press run)			717	663
b. Paid Circulation (By Mail and Outside the Mail)	(1)	Mailed Outside-County Paid Subscriptions Stated on PS Form 3541. (Include paid distribution above nominal rate, advertiser's proof copies, and exchange copies)	407	357
	(2)	Mailed In-County Paid Subscriptions Stated on PS Form 3541 (Include paid distribution above nominal rate, advertiser's proof copies, and exchange copies)		
	(3)	Paid Distribution Outside the Mails Including Sales Through Dealers and Carriers, Street Vendors, Counter Sales, and Other Paid Distribution Outside USPS®	76	75
	(4)	Paid Distribution by Other Classes Mailed Through the USPS (e.g. First-Class Mail®)		
c. Total Paid Distribution (Sum of 15b (1), (2), (3), and (4))			483	432
d. Free or Nominal Rate Distribution (By Mail and Outside the Mail)	(1)	Free or Nominal Rate Outside-County Copies Included on PS Form 3541	117	141
	(2)	Free or Nominal Rate In-County Copies Included on PS Form 3541		
	(3)	Free or Nominal Rate Copies Mailed at Other Classes Through the USPS (e.g. First-Class Mail)		
	(4)	Free or Nominal Rate Distribution Outside the Mail (Carriers or other means)		
e. Total Free or Nominal Rate Distribution (Sum of 15d (1), (2), (3) and (4))			117	141
f. Total Distribution (Sum of 15c and 15e)			600	573
g. Copies not Distributed (See Instructions to publishers #4 (page 3))			117	90
h. Total (Sum of 15f and g)			717	663
i. Percent Paid (15c divided by 15f times 100)			80.50%	75.39%

16 Total circulation includes electronic copies. Report circulation on PS Form 3526-X worksheet.

17. Publication of Statement of Ownership
If the publication is a general publication, publication of this statement is required. Will be printed in the **October 2014** issue of this publication.

18. Signature and Title of Editor, Publisher, Business Manager, or Owner	Date
Stephen R. Bushing – Inventory Distribution Coordinator	September 14, 2014

I certify that all information furnished on this form is true and complete. I understand that anyone who furnishes false or misleading information on this form or who omits material or information requested on the form may be subject to criminal sanctions (including fines and imprisonment) and/or civil sanctions (including civil penalties).

PS Form 3526, August 2012 (Page 2 of 3)

Moving?

Make sure your subscription moves with you!

To notify us of your new address, find your **Clinics Account Number** (located on your mailing label above your name), and contact customer service at:

Email: journalscustomerservice-usa@elsevier.com

800-654-2452 (subscribers in the U.S. & Canada)
314-447-8871 (subscribers outside of the U.S. & Canada)

Fax number: 314-447-8029

Elsevier Health Sciences Division
Subscription Customer Service
3251 Riverport Lane
Maryland Heights, MO 63043

*To ensure uninterrupted delivery of your subscription, please notify us at least 4 weeks in advance of move.

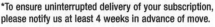

Printed and bound by CPI Group (UK) Ltd, Croydon, CR0 4YY

07/10/2024

01040498-0002